Student Workbook

Essentials of Dental Assisting

Seventh Edition

Student Workbook

Essentials of Dental Assisting

Seventh Edition

Debbie S. Robinson, CDA, MS
Retired
Dental Assisting
University of North Carolina
Chapel Hill, NC, United States

ELSEVIER

Elsevier
3251 Riverport Lane
St. Louis, Missouri 63043

STUDENT WORKBOOK FOR ESSENTIALS OF DENTAL ASSISTING, SEVENTH EDITION

ISBN: 978-0-323-77812-1

Notice

Practitioners and researchers must always rely on their own experience and knowledge in evaluating and using any information, methods, compounds or experiments described herein. Because of rapid advances in the medical sciences, in particular, independent verification of diagnoses and drug dosages should be made. To the fullest extent of the law, no responsibility is assumed by Elsevier, authors, editors or contributors for any injury and/or damage to persons or property as a matter of products liability, negligence or otherwise, or from any use or operation of any methods, products, instructions, or ideas contained in the material herein.

Previous editions copyrighted 2017, 2013, and 2007.

Content Strategist: Joslyn Dumas/Kelly Skelton
Senior Content Development Manager: Luke Held
Senior Content Development Specialist: Maria Broeker
Publishing Services Manager: Deepthi Unni
Project Manager: Thoufiq Mohammed
Design Direction: Gopalakrishnan Venkatraman

Printed in India

Last digit is the print number: 9 8 7 6 5 4 3 2 1

Working together to grow libraries in developing countries

www.elsevier.com • www.bookaid.org

Introduction

The student workbook is designed to help you prepare for and master the preclinical and clinical procedures presented in *Essentials of Dental Assisting*, Seventh Edition. The design allows the pages to be easily removed and submitted if required for a specific class. The workbook includes the following:

CHAPTER EXERCISES

Chapters include a variety of exercises, such as short answer questions, which come from the chapter's learning outcomes; fill-in-the-blank and matching questions, which are from the key terms of the chapter; and multiple-choice questions to reinforce the chapter content.

The chapter exercises are intended to help you study and prepare for a class, lab, or preclinic setting and to better understand the information presented in the corresponding chapter of the textbook. Please take the time to work through them carefully. Answers to the workbook exercises are available through your instructor.

COMPETENCY SHEETS

A competency is the process that is used to evaluate the dental assistant's mastery of preclinical, clinical, and advanced skills. The competency sheets included within this workbook are designed to give you the opportunity to practice a skill until you have mastered it. There are spaces on the form that allow for at least three different evaluations: from yourself, from a peer, and from your instructor. The first time you perform a competency, you may wish to evaluate your own performance. The second time, you might ask a classmate to give you feedback. When you feel comfortable with that skill, the evaluator would be your instructor, clinic supervisor, or dentist.

FLASHCARDS

The flashcards located in the back of the workbook can be easily removed and become a bonus study tool. The flashcards are selected from key information throughout the textbook and include the sciences, medical emergencies, infection control, radiography, dental materials, instruments, and dental procedures to help you prepare for courses and also for the Dental Assisting National Board and State Certification exams.

We wish you success in your studies and in your chosen profession of dental assisting.

Debbie S. Robinson

Contents

1 Introduction to Dental Assisting

TRUE/FALSE

_____ 1. Evidence of decay in human teeth has been detected since ancient times.

_____ 2. The most important person in the dental practice is the patient.

_____ 3. The dental laboratory technician completes his or her work according to a prescription written by the dental assistant.

_____ 4. The circulating assistant is used in four-handed dentistry.

_____ 5. A dental hygienist must pass both a written and a clinical examination to become licensed.

_____ 6. As of 2020, the ADA recognizes eight dental specialties.

_____ 7. The first dentist to use a dental assistant was Dr. C. Edmund Kells.

SHORT ANSWER

List the members of the dental health team.

8.

9.

10.

11.

List the dental specialties.

12.

13.

14.

15.

16.

17.

18.

19.

20.

21.

22.

List and describe the functionality of each area found in a dental office.

23.

24.

25.

26.

27.

28.

FILL IN THE BLANK

29. _____ is the specialty concerned with the diagnosis and surgical treatment of disorders, injuries, and defects of the oral and maxillofacial region.

30. _____ is the specialty focused on the diagnosis and treatment of diseases of the supporting and surrounding tissues of the teeth.

31. _____ is the specialty focused on the correction of malocclusion of the teeth and associated structures.

32. _____ is the specialty focused on the prevention and control of dental diseases and promotion of dental health through organized community efforts.

33. _____ specializes in the preventive and oral healthcare of children from birth through adolescence.

34. _____ is the specialty concerned with the diagnosis, prevention, and treatment of diseases and injuries of the pulp and associated structures.

35. _____ is the specialty concerned with the nature of diseases affecting the oral cavity and adjacent structures.

36. _____ is the specialty concerned with restoration and maintenance of oral functions by the restoration of natural teeth and/or replacement of missing teeth.

2 Professional and Legal Aspects of Dental Assisting

SHORT ANSWER

List three steps for good risk management.

1.

2.

3.

Give three essential aspects of a professional appearance.

4.

5.

6.

List four personal qualities of a good dental assistant.

7.

8.

9.

10.

FILL IN THE BLANK

11. _____ is when the dentist is physically present in the office at the time the auxiliary performs certain functions.

12. _____ involves codes of behavior, values, and morals.

13. _____ is the agency responsible for reviewing chemical use in the dental office.

14. _____ is the organization that addresses issues of infection control.

15. The _____ ensures that all dental and medical devices are safe and effective.

16. _____ is when the dentist does not have to be physically present when the dental auxiliary performs certain functions.

17. _____ is the agency responsible for employee safety.

18. A statement made at the time of an alleged negligent act and that is admissible as evidence in a court of law is called _____.

MULTIPLE CHOICE QUESTIONS

19. The patient record is important for which of the following reasons:
    a. All documents, images, and correspondence related to the patient are present
    b. Complete patient records are valuable in court if there were to be a malpractice case
    c. The record clearly shows dates and details of services
    d. All of the above

20. Which of the following statement(s) is *true* concerning types of law in the dental office?
    a. A dental assistant is in violation of criminal law if they perform a dental procedure that is not legal for them to perform in their state
    b. A dentist is in violation of criminal law if they commit insurance fraud
    c. A patient can sue a dentist based on inadequate treatment, resulting in a civil lawsuit
    d. All of the above

21. Which of the following statement(s) in ownership of dental records and radiographs is *true*?
    a. The dentist "owns" all patient records and radiographs.
    b. Patients have a right to review their records and radiographs.
    c. Original records and radiographs should never be allowed to leave the practice without the permission of the dentist.
    d. All of the above

22. Which of the following statements is *not true* regarding consent?
    a. Informed consent occurs when the patient and dentist discuss all options available to the patient and then the patient chooses the most suitable option
    b. Implied consent occurs when a dentist provides a treatment that they believe is necessary for the patient
    c. Written consent is preferred when obtaining a patient's consent and understanding of a procedure
    d. Implied consent is the least reliable form of consent in a malpractice suit

23. Which of the following statement(s) regarding informed consent for minors is true?
    a. If parents are separated, then it is appropriate to send records to a designated parent
    b. Blanket consent is beneficial because it allows for dentists to provide emergency care when a parent or guardian is not present
    c. A child's personal form should not include personal details regarding parental separation
    d. None of the above

24. The main objective of the State Dental Practice Act is to:
    a. Regulate dental practice cleanliness
    b. Protect the public from incompetent dental health care providers
    c. Protect dental practice privacy
    d. Ensure that dental practices cannot be sued

25. Which of the following statement(s) about the State Board of Dentistry is *true*?
    a. The board has the authority to issue, revoke, suspend, or deny renewal of licenses
    b. The board outlines reciprocity agreements between states
    c. The members of the board are appointed by the governor of the state
    d. All of the above

3 Anatomy and Physiology

TRUE/FALSE

_____ 1. The midsagittal plane is the plane that divides the human body into equal left and right halves.

_____ 2. Cells are the smallest living unit of the human body.

_____ 3. Tissues in the human body are groups of specialized cells that join to perform a specific function.

_____ 4. A frenum is a narrow band of tissue that connects two bones.

_____ 5. The trigeminal nerve is the primary source of innervation for the oral cavity.

_____ 6. There are three primary types of tissue found in the human body.

_____ 7. The TMJ makes it possible for the mandible to move.

_____ 8. The temporal process of the zygomatic bone forms the back of the skull.

_____ 9. The occipital bone forms the chin.

_____ 10. The frontal bone forms the forehead.

11. Below is a list of the major body systems. Provide the major functions and make-up of each system:
   a. Skeletal
   b. Muscular
   c. Cardiovascular
   d. Lymphatic and Immune
   e. Nervous
   f. Respiratory
   g. Digestive
   h. Urinary
   i. Integumentary
   j. Endocrine
   k. Reproductive

LABELING

12. Label the bones and landmarks of the hard palate.

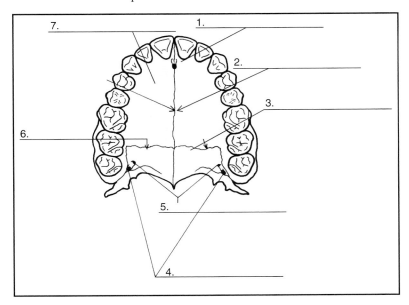

13. Label the salivary glands.

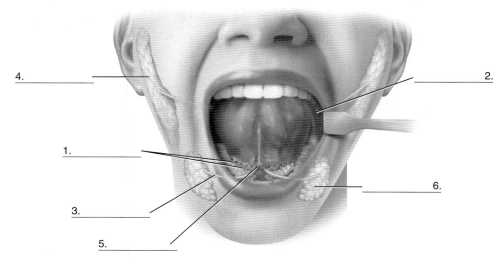

©Elsevier collection

14. Label the topical view of the mandible.

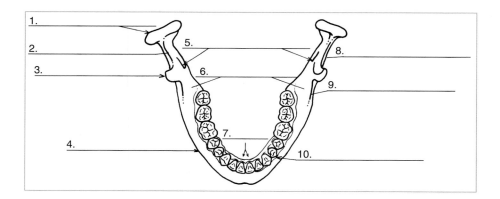

COMPETENCY 3-1 IDENTIFY THE MAJOR LANDMARKS AND STRUCTURES OF THE FACE

Performance Objective

By following a routine procedure that meets stated protocols, the student will be able to correctly identify the major landmarks and structures of the face.

Evaluation and Grading Criteria

3   Student competently met the stated criteria without assistance.

2   Student required assistance to meet the stated criteria.

1   Student showed uncertainty when performing the stated criteria.

0   Student was not prepared and needs to repeat the step.

N/A   No evaluation of this step.

Instructor shall define grades for each point range earned upon completion of each performance-evaluated task.

Performance Standards

The minimum number of satisfactory performances required prior to final evaluation is _____.

Instructor shall identify by * those steps considered critical. If step is missed or minimum competency is not met, the evaluated procedure fails and must be repeated.

Performance Criteria	*	Self	Peer	Instructor	Comments
1. Identifies the ala of the nose.					
2. Identifies the inner canthus and outer canthus of the eye.					
3. Identifies the commissure of the lips.					
4. Identifies the location of the frontal sinuses.					
5. Identifies the location of the maxillary sinuses.					
6. Identifies the location of the parotid glands.					
7. Identifies the philtrum.					
8. Identifies the tragus of the ear.					
9. Identifies the vermilion border.					
10. Identifies the zygomatic arch.					

Additional Comments

Total number of points possible _____

Total number of points received _____

Grade _____ *Instructor's initials* _____ *Date* _____

7

COMPETENCY 3-2 IDENTIFY THE MAJOR LANDMARKS, STRUCTURES, AND NORMAL TISSUES OF THE MOUTH

Performance Objective

By following a routine procedure that meets stated protocols, the student will be able to correctly identify the major landmarks, structures, and normal tissues of the mouth.

Evaluation and Grading Criteria

3   Student competently met the stated criteria without assistance.

2   Student required assistance to meet the stated criteria.

1   Student showed uncertainty when performing the stated criteria.

0   Student was not prepared and needs to repeat the step.

N/A   No evaluation of this step.

Instructor shall define grades for each point range earned upon completion of each performance-evaluated task.

Performance Standards

The minimum number of satisfactory performances required prior to final evaluation is _____.

Instructor shall identify by ∗ those steps considered critical. If step is missed or minimum competency is not met, the evaluated procedure fails and must be repeated.

Performance Criteria	∗	Self	Peer	Instructor	Comments
1. Identifies the dorsum of the tongue.					
2. Identifies the area of the gag reflex.					
3. Identifies the hard and soft palates.					
4. Identifies the gingival margin.					
5. Identifies the incisive papilla.					
6. Identifies the mandibular labial frenum.					
7. Identifies the maxillary labial frenum.					
8. Identifies the sublingual frenum.					
9. Identifies the vestibule of the mouth.					
10. Identifies Wharton's duct.					
Additional Comments					

Total number of points possible _____

Total number of points received _____

Grade _____ *Instructor's initials* _____ *Date* _____

4 Dental Anatomy

TRUE/FALSE

_____ 1. The clinical crown is the portion of the tooth that is visible in the mouth.

_____ 2. In the permanent dentition, there are 12 molar teeth.

_____ 3. An embrasure is the space between the roots of a molar.

_____ 4. Primary teeth are also known as deciduous teeth.

_____ 5. The anatomic crown is the portion of the tooth that is covered with enamel.

_____ 6. Bifurcation means division into three roots.

_____ 7. Molars and premolars have incisal surfaces.

_____ 8. Dentin makes up the main portion of the tooth structure.

_____ 9. Cementum is harder than enamel or dentin.

_____ 10. Only posterior teeth have periodontal ligaments.

LABELING

11. Label the tissues of the tooth and surrounding structures.

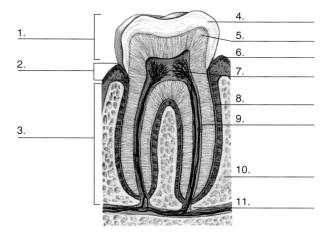

1. _____
2. _____
3. _____
4. _____
5. _____
6. _____
7. _____
8. _____
9. _____
10. _____
11. _____

12. Using the universal numbering system, number the teeth in the diagram below:

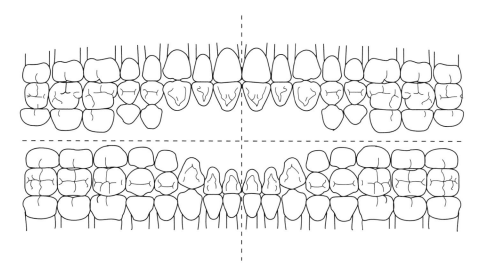

13. Label the surfaces of the teeth:

1. _____

2. _____

3. _____

4. _____

5. _____

6. _____

7. _____

8. _____

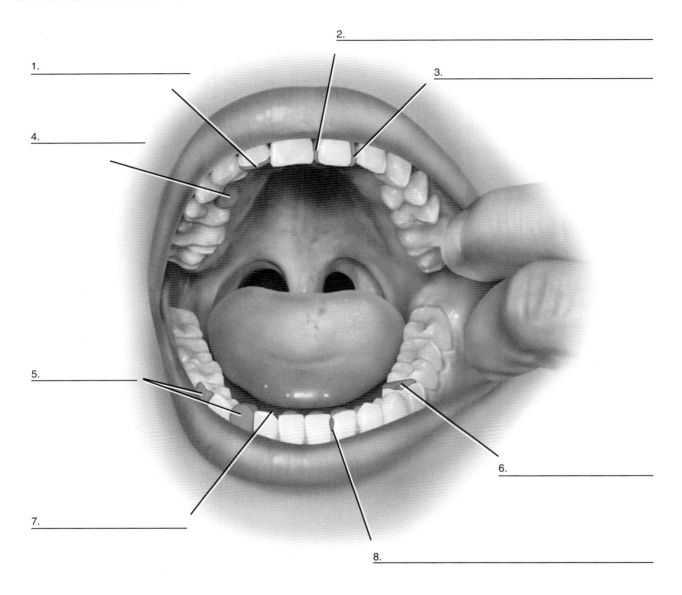

©Elsevier collection

COMPETENCY 4-1 IDENTIFY THE TEETH AND NAME THE TOOTH SURFACES

Performance Objective

By following a routine procedure that meets stated protocols, the student will be able to correctly identify the teeth and name the tooth surfaces.

Evaluation and Grading Criteria

3   Student competently met the stated criteria without assistance.

2   Student required assistance in order to meet the stated criteria.

1   Student showed uncertainty when performing the stated criteria.

0   Student was not prepared and needs to repeat the step.

N/A   No evaluation of this step.

Instructor shall define grades for each point range earned upon completion of each performance-evaluated task.

Performance Standards

The minimum number of satisfactory performances required prior to final evaluation is _____.

Instructor shall identify by ∗ those steps considered critical. If step is missed or minimum competency is not met, the evaluated procedure fails and must be repeated.

Performance Criteria	∗	Self	Peer	Instructor	Comments
1. Identifies the maxillary central incisors.					
2. Identifies the mandibular central incisors.					
3. Identifies the maxillary lateral incisors.					
4. Identifies the mandibular lateral incisors.					
5. Identifies the maxillary canines.					
6. Identifies the mandibular canines.					
7. Identifies the maxillary premolars.					
8. Identifies the mandibular premolars.					
9. Identifies the maxillary molars.					
10. Identifies the mandibular molars.					
11. Identifies the occlusal surfaces.					
12. Identifies the incisal surfaces.					
13. Identifies the lingual surfaces.					
14. Identifies the facial surfaces.					
15. Identifies the mesial surface of the maxillary central incisors.					
16. Identifies the distal surface of the mandibular central incisors.					
Additional Comments					

Chapter **4** **Dental Anatomy**

Total number of points possible _____

Total number of points received _____

Grade _____ *Instructor's initials* _____ *Date* _____

COMPETENCY 4-2 IDENTIFY THE PRIMARY AND PERMANENT DENTITIONS USING THE UNIVERSAL NATIONAL SYSTEM, THE FEDERATION DENTAIRE INTERNATIONALE SYSTEM, AND THE PALMER NOTATION SYSTEM

Performance Objective

By following a routine procedure that meets stated protocols, the student will be able to correctly identify the teeth using each of the numbering systems.

Evaluation and Grading Criteria

3   Student competently met the stated criteria without assistance.

2   Student required assistance in order to meet the stated criteria.

1   Student showed uncertainty when performing the stated criteria.

0   Student was not prepared and needs to repeat the step.

N/A   No evaluation of this step.

Instructor shall define grades for each point range earned upon completion of each performance-evaluated task.

Performance Standards

The minimum number of satisfactory performances required prior to final evaluation is _____.

Instructor shall identify by ∗ those steps considered critical. If step is missed or minimum competency is not met, the evaluated procedure fails and must be repeated.

Performance Criteria	∗	Self	Peer	Instructor	Comments
1. Identifies the primary teeth in each arch using the Universal/National System.					
2. Identifies the primary teeth in each arch using the Federation Dentaire Internationale Numbering System.					
3. Identifies the primary teeth in each arch using the Palmer Notation System.					
4. Identifies the permanent teeth in each arch using the Universal System.					
5. Identifies the permanent teeth in each arch using the Federation Dentaire Internationale Numbering System.					
6. Identifies the permanent teeth in each arch using the Palmer Notation System.					

Additional Comments

Total number of points possible _____

Total number of points received _____

Grade _____ *Instructor's initials* _____ *Date* _____

15

5 Microbiology and Disease Transmission

TRUE/FALSE

_____ 1. A pathogen is a microorganism that is not capable of causing disease.

_____ 2. Many types of bacteria are actually beneficial to humans.

_____ 3. When bacteria are in the spore state, they cannot cause disease.

_____ 4. Viruses are much larger than bacteria.

_____ 5. Virulence describes the ability of a pathogen to cause disease.

_____ 6. An acute infection is of short duration.

_____ 7. Indirect transmission of disease is also known as *cross-contamination.*

_____ 8. Diseases cannot be transmitted during a dental procedure through aerosol or spray throughout a procedure.

_____ 9. Airborne disease transmission is also known as *droplet infection.*

_____ 10. The term *parenteral transmission* refers to disease spread from parent to child.

FILL IN THE BLANK

11. The number of pathogens present is called the _____.

12. _____ is a disease caused by a spore-forming bacillus.

13. The ability of the human body to resist disease is called _____.

14. The method by which the pathogen enters the body is called the _____.

15. Plants yeasts, and molds are examples of _____.

16. _____ is a disease of the liver with a latency of up to 15 to 25 years.

17. _____ is a disease of the liver caused by fecal-oral transmission.

18. _____ is a type of disease normally caused by nonpathogenic organisms.

19. _____ is a disease caused by the yeast *Candida albicans.*

20. _____ transmission occurs through a break in the skin.

MULTIPLE CHOICE

21. Which of the following organisms live and multiply only inside a host cell?
    a. bacteria
    b. virus
    c. spore
    d. all of the above

22. The links in the chain of infection include the infectious agent, reservoir, portal of exit, transmission, portal of entry and _____.
    a. latency
    b. host susceptibility
    c. Infection
    d. pathogen

23. Which of the following surfaces could be a potential source of disease transmission in a dental office?
    a. faucets
    b. instrument drawer handles
    c. dental instrument
    d. the patient's chart
    e. all of the above

24. Dental aerosols can contain _____.
    a. saliva
    b. blood
    c. microorganisms
    d. all of the above

25. Which of the following are considered types of parenteral disease transmission?
    a. needle sticks
    b. human bites
    c. cuts
    d. all of the above

17

6 Infection Control and Management of Hazardous Materials

TRUE/FALSE

_____ 1. The Centers for Disease Control and Prevention (CDC) is not a regulatory agency.

_____ 2. OSHA's Bloodborne Pathogen Standard (BBP) is the most important infection-control law in dentistry.

_____ 3. The concept of "universal precautions" has been expanded, and the term for the new concept is "standard precautions."

_____ 4. A category III employee is routinely exposed to blood, saliva, or both.

_____ 5. The employer is not required to offer the hepatitis B vaccine to category III employees.

_____ 6. You should always bend or break needles before disposal.

_____ 7. The sharps container must be labeled with the biohazard symbol.

_____ 8. Alcohol-based hand rubs are not to be used if your hands are visibly soiled.

_____ 9. Artificial nails should not be worn by dental assistants.

_____ 10. Short-sleeve scrub tops are adequate protection when assisting in a clinical procedure.

FILL IN THE BLANK

11. A category _____ employee is one who is routinely exposed to blood and/or saliva.

12. Employers are required by the _____ _____ standard to provide employees with personal protective equipment.

13. A _____ is an acceptable alternative to eyewear.

14. _____ gloves are required for surgical procedures.

15. _____ gloves should be worn when disinfecting surfaces in the treatment room.

MULTIPLE CHOICE

16. The term "medical waste" refers to:
    a. contaminated waste
    b. infectious waste
    c. regulated waste
    d. all of the above

17. Which of the following must be included in a Hazard Communication program?
    a. written program
    b. chemical inventory
    c. safety data sheets
    d. employee training
    e. all of the above

18. The current OSHA Hazard Communication Standard has adopted which standard:
    a. Globally Harmonized System of Classification and Labeling of Chemicals
    b. Centers for Disease Control and Prevention Recommendations
    c. Federal Drug Administration Labeling System
    d. All of the above

19. According to OSHA's Hazard Communication Standard, records of employee's training must be kept on file a minimum of _____
    a. 1 year
    b. 3 years
    c. 5 years
    d. indefinitely

20. Which of the following are bloodborne pathogens?
    a. hepatitis B
    b. hepatitis C
    c. HIV
    d. all of the above

COMPETENCY 6-1 FIRST AID AFTER AN EXPOSURE INCIDENT

Performance Objective

By following a routine procedure that meets stated protocols, the student will be able to perform appropriate first aid after an exposure incident.

Evaluation and Grading Criteria

3	Student competently met the stated criteria without assistance.
2	Student required assistance to meet the stated criteria.
1	Student showed uncertainty when performing the stated criteria.
0	Student was not prepared and needs to repeat the step.
N/A	No evaluation of this step.

Instructor shall define grades for each point range earned upon completion of each performance-evaluated task.

Performance Standards

The minimum number of satisfactory performances required prior to final evaluation is _____.

Instructor shall identify by ∗ those steps considered critical. If step is missed or minimum competency is not met, the evaluated procedure fails and must be repeated.

Performance Criteria	∗	Self	Peer	Instructor	Comments
Stop Operations Immediately					
1. Removes gloves.					
2. Washes hands thoroughly, using antimicrobial soap and warm water.					
3. Dries hands.					
Apply a Small Amount of Antiseptic to the Affected Area					
4. Applies an adhesive bandage to the area.					
5. Completes applicable postexposure follow-up paperwork.					
Additional Comments					

Total number of points possible _____

Total number of points received _____

Grade _____ *Instructor's initials* _____ *Date* _____

21

Performance Objective

By following a routine procedure that meets stated protocols, the student will be able to wash hands properly before gloving.

Evaluation and Grading Criteria

3	Student competently met the stated criteria without assistance.
2	Student required assistance to meet the stated criteria.
1	Student showed uncertainty when performing the stated criteria.
0	Student was not prepared and needs to repeat the step.
N/A	No evaluation of this step.

Instructor shall define grades for each point range earned upon completion of each performance-evaluated task.

Performance Standards

The minimum number of satisfactory performances required prior to final evaluation is _____.

Instructor shall identify by ∗ those steps considered critical. If step is missed or minimum competency is not met, the evaluated procedure fails and must be repeated.

Performance Criteria	∗	Self	Peer	Instructor	Comments
1. Removes all jewelry, including watch and rings.					
2. Uses the foot or electronic control to regulate water flow. If this is not available, uses a paper towel to grasp the faucets to turn them on and off. Discards the towel after use. Allows hands to become wet.					
3. Applies soap; lathers using a circular motion with friction while holding fingertips downward. Rubs well between fingers. If this was the first handwashing of the day, uses a nailbrush or an orange stick. Inspects and cleans under every fingernail during this step.					
4. Vigorously rubs together the lathered hands under a stream of water to remove surface debris.					
5. Applies more soap and vigorously rubs together lathered hands for a minimum of 10 seconds under a stream of water.					
6. Rinses the hands with cool water.					
7. Uses a paper towel to dry the hands thoroughly and then dry the forearms.					
8. If water faucets are not foot operated, turns off the faucet with a clean paper towel.					
Additional Comments					

Total number of points possible _____

Total number of points received _____

Grade _____ Instructor's initials _____ Date _____

COMPETENCY 6-3 APPLYING ALCOHOL-BASED HAND RUBS

Performance Objective

By following a routine procedure that meets stated protocols, the student will be able to apply an alcohol-based hand rub.

Evaluation and Grading Criteria

3	Student competently met the stated criteria without assistance.
2	Student required assistance in order to meet the stated criteria.
1	Student showed uncertainty when performing the stated criteria.
0	Student was not prepared and needs to repeat the step.
N/A	No evaluation of this step.

Instructor shall define grades for each point range earned upon completion of each performance-evaluated task.

Performance Standards

The minimum number of satisfactory performances required prior to final evaluation is _____.

Instructor shall identify by * those steps considered critical. If step is missed or minimum competency is not met, the evaluated procedure fails and must be repeated.

Performance Criteria	*	Self	Peer	Instructor	Comments
1. Checks hands to be sure they are not visibly soiled or contaminated with organic matter, such as blood or saliva. If necessary, washes hands with soap and water and dries them thoroughly.					
2. Reads directions carefully to determine the proper amount to dispense.					
3. Dispenses the proper amount of the product into the palm of one hand.					
4. Rubs the palms of the hands together.					
5. Rubs the product between the fingers.					
6. Rubs the product over the back of the hands.					
Additional Comments					

Total number of points possible _____

Total number of points received _____

Grade _____ Instructor's initials _____ Date _____

Chapter **6** **Infection Control and Management of Hazardous Materials**

COMPETENCY 6-4 PUTTING ON PERSONAL PROTECTIVE EQUIPMENT (PPE)

Performance Objective

By following a routine procedure that meets stated protocols, the student will be able to put on personal protective equipment before patient care.

Evaluation and Grading Criteria

3   Student competently met the stated criteria without assistance.

2   Student required assistance in order to meet the stated criteria.

1   Student showed uncertainty when performing the stated criteria.

0   Student was not prepared and needs to repeat the step.

N/A   No evaluation of this step.

Instructor shall define grades for each point range earned upon completion of each performance-evaluated task.

Performance Standards

The minimum number of satisfactory performances required prior to final evaluation is _____.

Instructor shall identify by * those steps considered critical. If step is missed or minimum competency is not met, the evaluated procedure fails and must be repeated.

Performance Criteria	*	Self	Peer	Instructor	Comments
1. Places protective clothing over uniform, street clothes, or scrubs.					
2. Places surgical mask and adjusts the fit.					
3. Places protective eyewear.					
4. Thoroughly washes and dries hands.					
5. Holds one glove at the cuff, places opposite hand inside the glove and pulls it onto the hand. Repeats with a new glove for the other hand.					

Additional Comments

Total number of points possible _____

Total number of points received _____

Grade _____ Instructor's initials _____ Date _____

     Chapter **6**   **Infection Control and Management of Hazardous Materials**

COMPETENCY 6-5 REMOVING PERSONAL PROTECTIVE EQUIPMENT

Performance Objective

By following a routine procedure that meets stated protocols, the student will be able to remove personal protective equipment.

Evaluation and Grading Criteria

3	Student competently met the stated criteria without assistance.
2	Student required assistance in order to meet the stated criteria.
1	Student showed uncertainty when performing the stated criteria.
0	Student was not prepared and needs to repeat the step.
N/A	No evaluation of this step.

Instructor shall define grades for each point range earned upon completion of each performance-evaluated task.

Performance Standards

The minimum number of satisfactory performances required prior to final evaluation is _____.

Instructor shall identify by * those steps considered critical. If step is missed or minimum competency is not met, the evaluated procedure fails and must be repeated.

Performance Criteria	*	Self	Peer	Instructor	Comments
1. Uses gloved hand to grasp the other glove at the outside cuff. Pulls downward, turning the glove inside out as it is pulled away from hand.					
2. For the other hand, uses the ungloved fingers and grasps the inside (uncontaminated area) of the cuff of the remaining glove. Pulls downward to remove the glove, and turns it inside out. Discards the gloves into the waste receptacle.					
3. Washes and thoroughly dries hands.					
Eyewear					
1. Removes eyewear by touching it only on the ear rests (which were not contaminated).					
2. Places the eyewear on a disposable towel until it can be properly cleaned and disinfected.					
Mask					
1. Slides the fingers of each hand under the elastic strap in front of the ears and removes the mask. Discards the mask into the waste receptacle.					
Protective Clothing					
1. Pulls the gown off, turning it inside out as it comes off.					
Additional Comments					

Total number of points possible _____

Total number of points received _____

Grade _____ Instructor's initials _____ Date _____

Chapter **6** **Infection Control and Management of Hazardous Materials**

7 Surface Disinfection and Treatment Room Preparation

TRUE/FALSE

_____ 1. The purpose of surface barriers is to prevent contamination.

_____ 2. Only surfaces touched by the patient should be precleaned before disinfecting.

_____ 3. Utility gloves should be worn when precleaning surfaces.

_____ 4. Surfaces that are smooth and easily accessible are the easiest to clean and disinfect.

_____ 5. Precleaning is completed after the disinfection process.

_____ 6. Blood and saliva are also known as bioburden.

_____ 7. A contaminated surface must be disinfected.

_____ 8. Surface barriers should be resistant to fluids.

_____ 9. There is a variety of barriers used for infection control.

_____ 10. Not all types of disinfectants contain a precleaning agent.

FILL IN THE BLANK

11. Surgical forceps are classified as a _____ instrument.

12. An X-ray position indicating device (PID) is classified as a _____ instrument.

13. Sodium hypochlorite is classified as a _____ disinfectant.

14. The control buttons on the dental chair should be protected with a _____.

15. A _____ is the type of chemical to be used on contertops and equipment.

MULTIPLE CHOICE

16. Which of the following can be used as surface barriers?
    a. plastic bags
    b. aluminum foil
    c. plastic sticky tape
    d. all of the above

17. Which agency registers surface disinfectants?
    a. Environmental Protection Agency (EPA)
    b. Occupational Safety and Health Administration (OSHA)
    c. Food and Drug Administration (FDA)
    d. All of the above

18. Which of the following disinfectants can cause red or yellow stains?
    a. synthetic phenols
    b. iodophors
    c. sodium hypochlorite
    d. none of the above

19. Which of the following is a disadvantage of using alcohol as a disinfectant?
    a. rapid evaporation
    b. not effective in the presence of bioburden
    c. damaging to plastics and vinyl
    d. all of the above

20. Which of the following can be used as a high-level disinfectant or a sterilant?
    a. alcohol
    b. synthetic phenol
    c. glutaraldehyde
    d. all of the above

Performance Objective

By following a routine procedure that meets stated protocols, the student will be able to place surface barriers before patient treatment and remove the barriers at the end of the procedure.

Evaluation and Grading Criteria

3	Student competently met the stated criteria without assistance.
2	Student required assistance in order to meet the stated criteria.
1	Student showed uncertainty when performing the stated criteria.
0	Student was not prepared and needs to repeat the step.
N/A	No evaluation of this step.

Instructor shall define grades for each point range earned upon completion of each performance-evaluated task.

Performance Standards

The minimum number of satisfactory performances required prior to final evaluation is _____.

Instructor shall identify by * those steps considered critical. If step is missed or minimum competency is not met, the evaluated procedure fails and must be repeated.

Performance Criteria	*	Self	Peer	Instructor	Comments
1. Washes and dries hands.					
2. Selects the appropriate surface barrier to place over the clean surface.					
3. Places each barrier over the entire surface to be protected. Checks that the barrier is secure and will not come off.					
4. Wears utility gloves to remove contaminated surface barriers after dental treatment.					
5. Very carefully removes each cover without touching the underlying surface with either the utility glove or the contaminated outside surface of the barrier.					
6. Discards the used covers in the regular waste trash.					
7. Washes, disinfects, and removes utility gloves. Washes and dries hands, then applies fresh surface covers for the next patient.					

Additional Comments

Total number of points possible _____

Total number of points received _____

Grade _____ Instructor's initials _____ Date _____

Performance Objective

By following a routine procedure that meets stated protocols, the student will be able to clean and disinfect dental treatment rooms effectively.

Evaluation and Grading Criteria

3	Student competently met the stated criteria without assistance.
2	Student required assistance in order to meet the stated criteria.
1	Student showed uncertainty when performing the stated criteria.
0	Student was not prepared and needs to repeat the step.
N/A	No evaluation of this step.

Instructor shall define grades for each point range earned upon completion of each performance-evaluated task.

Performance Standards

The minimum number of satisfactory performances required prior to final evaluation is _____.

Instructor shall identify by * those steps considered critical. If step is missed or minimum competency is not met, the evaluated procedure fails and must be repeated.

Performance Criteria	*	Self	Peer	Instructor	Comments
1. Puts on utility gloves, protective eyewear, and protective clothing.					
2. Makes sure that the precleaning and/or disinfecting product is prepared correctly and is fresh. Makes certain to read and follow the manufacturer's instructions.					
3. To preclean, sprays the paper towel or gauze pad with the product and vigorously wipes the surface. Uses a small brush for surfaces that do not become visibly clean from wiping. If cleaning a large area, uses several towels or gauze pads.					
4. To disinfect, sprays a fresh paper towel or gauze pad with product. Allows the surface to remain moist for the manufacturer's recommended time (for tuberculocidal action, usually 10 minutes).					
5. If the surface is still moist after the kill time and must be ready to seat another patient, wipes the surface dry. Uses water to rinse any residual disinfectant from surfaces that will come in contact with the patient's skin or mouth.					
Additional Comments					

Total number of points possible _____

Total number of points received _____

Grade _____ *Instructor's initials* _____ *Date* _____

Chapter **7** **Surface Disinfection and Treatment Room Preparation**

8 Instrument Processing

TRUE/FALSE

_____ 1. The ideal instrument-processing center should be dedicated only to instrument processing.

_____ 2. An advantage of dry heat sterilization is that it does not corrode or rust instruments.

_____ 3. The sterilization center should be in a high-traffic area for easier access

_____ 4. The container of the holding solution should be labeled with a biohazard label and a chemical label.

_____ 5. Contaminated and sterile instruments may be stored in the same cabinet if they are packaged.

SHORT ANSWER

List the seven steps in instrument processing, briefly describe the purpose of each step.

6.

7.

8.

9.

10.

11.

12.

List three advantages of the steam autoclave.

13.

14.

15.

FILL IN THE BLANK

16. _____ is the least desirable method of precleaning instruments.

17. A _____ prevents blood and debris from drying on the instrument.

18. A _____ is used to lossen and remove debris from instruments.

19. An _____ sterilizes instruments by using super-heated steam under pressure.

20. An automated washing and disinfecting machine is classified as a _____.

COMPETENCY 8-1 OPERATING THE ULTRASONIC CLEANER

Performance Objective

By following a routine procedure that meets stated protocols, the student will be able to prepare and use the ultrasonic cleaner effectively.

Evaluation and Grading Criteria

3	Student competently met the stated criteria without assistance.
2	Student required assistance in order to meet the stated criteria.
1	Student showed uncertainty when performing the stated criteria.
0	Student was not prepared and needs to repeat the step.
N/A	No evaluation of this step.

Instructor shall define grades for each point range earned upon completion of each performance-evaluated task.

Performance Standards

The minimum number of satisfactory performances required prior to final evaluation is _____.

Instructor shall identify by * those steps considered critical. If step is missed or minimum competency is not met, the evaluated procedure fails and must be repeated.

Performance Criteria	*	Self	Peer	Instructor	Comments
1. Puts on protective clothing, mask, eyewear, and utility gloves.					
2. Removes the lid from the container.					
3. Confirms the container is filled with the solution to the level recommended by the manufacturer.					
4. Places loose instruments in the basket or, if using cassettes, places the cassette in the basket.					
5. Replaces the lid, and turns the cycle to "On."					
6. After the cleaning cycle, removes the basket and thoroughly rinses the instruments in a sink under tap water with minimal splashing. Holds the basket at an angle to allow water to run off into the sink to minimize splashing.					
7. Gently turns the basket onto a towel and removes the instruments or cassettes. Replaces the lid on the ultrasonic cleaner.					
Additional Comments					

Total number of points possible _____

Total number of points received _____

Grade _____ Instructor's initials _____ Date _____

Performance Objective

By following a routine procedure that meets stated protocols, the student will be able to prepare and autoclave instruments.

Evaluation and Grading Criteria

3   Student competently met the stated criteria without assistance.

2   Student required assistance in order to meet the stated criteria.

1   Student showed uncertainty when performing the stated criteria.

0   Student was not prepared and needs to repeat the step.

N/A   No evaluation of this step.

Instructor shall define grades for each point range earned upon completion of each performance-evaluated task.

Performance Standards

The minimum number of satisfactory performances required prior to final evaluation is _____.

Instructor shall identify by * those steps considered critical. If step is missed or minimum competency is not met, the evaluated procedure fails and must be repeated.

Performance Criteria	*	Self	Peer	Instructor	Comments
1. Cleans instruments before wrapping for autoclave.					
2. Dips nonstainless instruments and burs in a corrosion inhibitor solution before wrapping.					
3. Inserts the process integrator into the package.					
4. Packages, seals, and labels the instruments.					
Load the Autoclave 1. Places bagged and sealed items in the autoclave.					
2. Separates articles and packs from each other by a reasonable space. Tilted glass or metal canisters are positioned at an angle.					
3. Places packs in the chamber according to the manufacturer's recommendations.					
4. Does not overload the autoclave.					
Operate the Autoclave 1. Reads and follows the manufacturer's instructions.					
2. Ensures that an adequate supply of water is available. If not, adds distilled water.					
3. Sets autoclave controls for the appropriate time, temperature, and pressure.					
4. At the end of the sterilization cycle, vents the steam into the room. Allows the contents of the autoclave to dry and cool.					

Performance Criteria	*	Self	Peer	Instructor	Comments
Reassemble and Store the Trays 1. Washes hands and puts on clean examination gloves for handling sterile packs and reassembling trays.					
2. Removes sealed packs from the sterilizer and places them in the clean area.					
3. Places the sealed packs on the tray and adds the supplies necessary to perform the procedure.					
4. Stores the prepared tray in the clean area until needed in the treatment room.					
Additional Comments					

Total number of points possible _____

Total number of points received _____

Grade _____ *Instructor's initials* _____ *Date* _____

COMPETENCY 8-3 STERILIZING INSTRUMENTS WITH CHEMICAL VAPOR

Performance Objective

By following a routine procedure that meets stated protocols, the student will be able to prepare and sterilize instruments by chemical vapor sterilization.

Evaluation and Grading Criteria

3   Student competently met the stated criteria without assistance.

2   Student required assistance in order to meet the stated criteria.

1   Student showed uncertainty when performing the stated criteria.

0   Student was not prepared and needs to repeat the step.

N/A   No evaluation of this step.

Instructor shall define grades for each point range earned upon completion of each performance-evaluated task.

Performance Standards

The minimum number of satisfactory performances required prior to final evaluation is _____.

Instructor shall identify by * those steps considered critical. If step is missed or minimum competency is not met, the evaluated procedure fails and must be repeated.

Performance Criteria	*	Self	Peer	Instructor	Comments
Wrap the Instruments					
1. Ensures that the instruments are clean and dry before wrapping them for chemical vapor sterilization.					
2. Inserts the appropriate process integrator into the test load instrument package.					
3. Takes care not to prepare packs that are too large to be sterilized throughout.					
Load and Operate the Chemical Vapor Sterilizer					
1. Reads and follows the manufacturer's instructions.					
2. Loads the sterilizer according to the manufacturer's instructions.					
3. Sets the controls for the appropriate time, temperature, and pressure.					
4. Follows the manufacturer's instructions for venting and cooling.					
5. When the instruments are cool and dry, reassembles and stores the preset trays.					
Additional Comments					

Total number of points possible _____

Total number of points received _____

Grade _____ Instructor's initials _____ Date _____

43

Performance Objective

By following a routine procedure that meets stated protocols, the student will be able to prepare and sterilize instruments by dry heat sterilization.

Evaluation and Grading Criteria

3   Student competently met the stated criteria without assistance.

2   Student required assistance in order to meet the stated criteria.

1   Student showed uncertainty when performing the stated criteria.

0   Student was not prepared and needs to repeat the step.

N/A   No evaluation of this step.

Instructor shall define grades for each point range earned upon completion of each performance-evaluated task.

Performance Standards

The minimum number of satisfactory performances required prior to final evaluation is _____.

Instructor shall identify by * those steps considered critical. If step is missed or minimum competency is not met, the evaluated procedure fails and must be repeated.

Performance Criteria	*	Self	Peer	Instructor	Comments
Wrap Instruments					
1. Cleans and dries instruments before wrapping.					
2. Prepares hinged instruments, such as surgical forceps, hemostats, and scissors, with their hinges opened.					
Load and Operate the Dry Heat Sterilizer					
1. Reads and follows the manufacturer's instructions.					
2. Inserts the process integrator into the test load package.					
3. Loads the dry heat chamber to permit adequate circulation of air around the packages.					
4. Sets the time and temperature according to the manufacturer's instructions. Allows time for the entire load to reach the desired temperature.					
5. Does not place additional instruments in the load once the sterilization cycle has begun.					
6. At the end of the sterilization cycle, allows the packs to cool, then handles them very carefully.					
7. When the packs are cool, reassembles and stores the preset trays.					
Additional Comments					

Total number of points possible _____

Total number of points received _____

Grade _____ *Instructor's initials* _____ *Date* _____

45

COMPETENCY 8-5 STERILIZING INSTRUMENTS WITH CHEMICAL LIQUID

Performance Objective

By following a routine procedure that meets stated protocols, the student will be able to prepare and sterilize instruments using a chemical sterilant.

Evaluation and Grading Criteria

3   Student competently met the stated criteria without assistance.

2   Student required assistance in order to meet the stated criteria.

1   Student showed uncertainty when performing the stated criteria.

0   Student was not prepared and needs to repeat the step.

N/A   No evaluation of this step.

Instructor shall define grades for each point range earned upon completion of each performance-evaluated task.

Performance Standards

The minimum number of satisfactory performances required prior to final evaluation is _____.

Instructor shall identify by * those steps considered critical. If step is missed or minimum competency is not met, the evaluated procedure fails and must be repeated.

Performance Criteria	*	Self	Peer	Instructor	Comments
Prepare the Solution 1. Uses utility gloves, mask, eyewear, and protective clothing when preparing, using, and discarding the solution.					
2. Follows the manufacturer's instructions for preparing/activating, using, and disposing of the solution.					
3. Labels the containers with the name of the chemical, the date of preparation, and other information related to the hazards of the product.					
4. Covers the container and keeps it closed unless putting instruments in or taking them out.					
Use the Solution 1. Precleans, rinses, and dries items to be processed.					
2. Places the items in a perforated tray or pan. Places the pan in the solution and covers the container. Alternatively, uses tongs to avoid splashing.					
3. Is certain that all items were fully submerged in the solution for the entire contact time.					
4. Rinses processed items thoroughly with water and dries them. Places items in clean package.					

Performance Criteria	*	Self	Peer	Instructor	Comments
Maintain the Solution 1. Periodically tests the chemical liquid concentration of the solution with a chemical test kit.					
2. Replaces the solution as indicated on the instructions or when the level of the solution is low or the solution is visibly dirty.					
3. When replacing the used solution, discards all of the used solution, cleans the container with a detergent, rinses with water, dries, and fills with a fresh solution.					
Additional Comments					

Total number of points possible _____

Total number of points received _____

Grade _____ Instructor's initials _____ Date _____

COMPETENCY 8-6 PERFORMING BIOLOGIC MONITORING

Performance Objective

By following a routine procedure that meets stated protocols, the student will be able to assess sterilization using BIs (spore tests).

Evaluation and Grading Criteria

3   Student competently met the stated criteria without assistance.

2   Student required assistance in order to meet the stated criteria.

1   Student showed uncertainty when performing the stated criteria.

0   Student was not prepared and needs to repeat the step.

N/A   No evaluation of this step.

Instructor shall define grades for each point range earned upon completion of each performance-evaluated task.

Performance Standards

The minimum number of satisfactory performances required prior to final evaluation is _____.

Instructor shall identify by * those steps considered critical. If step is missed or minimum competency is not met, the evaluated procedure fails and must be repeated.

Performance Criteria	*	Self	Peer	Instructor	Comments
1. While wearing PPE, places the biologic indicator (BI) strip in the bundle of instruments and seals the package.					
2. Places the pack with the BI in the center of the sterilizer load.					
3. Places the remainder of the packaged instruments in the sterilizer and processes the load through a normal sterilization cycle.					
4. Removes utility gloves, mask, and eyewear. Washes and dries hands.					
5. In the sterilization log, records the date of the test, the type of the sterilizer, cycle, temperature, time, and the name of the person operating the sterilizer.					
6. After the load has been sterilized, removes the processed BI strip.					
7. Mails the processed spore test strips and the control BI to the monitoring service.					
Additional Comments					

Total number of points possible _____

Total number of points received _____

Grade _____ Instructor's initials _____ Date _____

9 The Dental Patient

TRUE/FALSE

_____ 1. A patient record is commonly referred to as the "patient's account."

_____ 2. The medical history update form should be completed, reviewed, and authorized with a signature to confirm the information provided.

_____ 3. Before a consultation can take place between a physician and dentist, the patient must sign a release of information form.

_____ 4. When taking a pulse reading, it is also important to note any changes in rhythm and depth.

_____ 5. A HIPAA policy should be in place and visible in every dental office.

_____ 6. Vital signs are indicators of a patient's overall health; they include temperature, pulse, weight, and blood pressure.

_____ 7. A patient's temperature is taken with a thermometer.

_____ 8. A patient has a blood pressure reading of 132/78; the second number is termed the systolic reading.

_____ 9. The instrument used to amplify the blood pumping through an artery is the sphygmomanometer.

_____ 10. A normal respiration rate for children is 10 to 20 breaths per minute.

MATCHING

_____ 11. The patient's past and present physical condition

_____ 12. A patient's agreement

_____ 13. Attention to drug sensitivities, allergic reactions, premedication's, or precautions

_____ 14. Indication for a change in a medical history

_____ 15. Treatment plan in a sequenced format

A. Dental problem list

B. Medical alert

C. Medical history update

D. Consent

E. Medical history

SHORT ANSWER

16. List three reasons for having a patient update their medical history at each appointment.

17. Identify the three most common locations to detect a patient's pulse and describe why and when these sites would be used.

18. What is the best advised sequence when taking a patient's vital signs?

19. List some of the more common allergies that should be noted in a patient record.

20. You are taking a blood pressure reading on a new patient. Because you do not have a previous reading, how do you know how high to pump the sphygmomanometer?

COMPETENCY 9-1 REGISTERING A NEW PATIENT

Performance Objective

By following a routine procedure that meets stated protocols, the student will be able to register a new patient.

Evaluation and Grading Criteria

3   Student competently met the stated criteria without assistance.

2   Student required assistance in order to meet the stated criteria.

1   Student showed uncertainty when performing the stated criteria.

0   Student was not prepared and needs to repeat the step.

N/A   No evaluation of this step.

Instructor shall define grades for each point range earned upon completion of each performance-evaluated task.

Performance Standards

The minimum number of satisfactory performances required prior to final evaluation is _____.

Instructor shall identify by * those steps considered critical. If step is missed or minimum competency is not met, the evaluated procedure fails and must be repeated.

Performance Criteria	*	Self	Peer	Instructor	Comments
1. Explains the need for the form to be completed. Provides the registration form, along with a clipboard and black pen.					
2. Reviews the completed form for the necessary information: a. Full name, birth date, and name of spouse or parent b. Home address and telephone number c. Occupation, name of employer, business address, and telephone number d. Name and address of person responsible for payment e. Method of payment (cash, check, credit, assignment of benefits) f. Health insurance information (photocopy of both sides of insurance ID card) g. Name of primary insurance carrier h. Group policy number					
3. Verifies that the patient has provided a signature and date on the form.					
Additional Comments					

Total number of points possible _____

Total number of points received _____

Grade _____ Instructor's initials _____ Date _____

COMPETENCY 9-2 OBTAINING A MEDICAL-DENTAL HEALTH HISTORY

Performance Objective

By following a routine procedure that meets stated protocols, the student will be able to obtain medical and dental health history information from a patient.

Evaluation and Grading Criteria

3   Student competently met the stated criteria without assistance.

2   Student required assistance in order to meet the stated criteria.

1   Student showed uncertainty when performing the stated criteria.

0   Student was not prepared and needs to repeat the step.

N/A   No evaluation of this step.

Instructor shall define grades for each point range earned upon completion of each performance-evaluated task.

Performance Standards

The minimum number of satisfactory performances required prior to final evaluation is _____.

Instructor shall identify by * those steps considered critical. If step is missed or minimum competency is not met, the evaluated procedure fails and must be repeated.

Performance Criteria	*	Self	Peer	Instructor	Comments
1. Explains the need for the information and the importance of fully completing the form.					
2. Provides the patient with a black pen and the form on a clipboard.					
3. Offers assistance to the patient in completing the form.					
4. Asks the patient to return the form and clipboard after answering all the questions.					
5. Thanks the patient for completing the form and requests that the patient take a seat in the reception area.					
6. Reviews the form for errors and/or any questions that may arise before handing it to the clinical assistant.					
7. Uses the information from the patient's medical-dental health history form to complete other documents. Notes that the information provided by the patient is confidential and must be maintained as such.					
Additional Comments					

Total number of points possible _____

Total number of points received _____

Grade _____ *Instructor's initials* _____ *Date* _____

55

COMPETENCY 9-3 TAKING AN ORAL TEMPERATURE READING WITH A DIGITAL THERMOMETER

Performance Objective

By following a routine procedure that meets stated protocols, the student will be able to take an oral temperature reading with a digital thermometer.

Evaluation and Grading Criteria

3 Student competently met the stated criteria without assistance.

2 Student required assistance in order to meet the stated criteria.

1 Student showed uncertainty when performing the stated criteria.

0 Student was not prepared and needs to repeat the step.

N/A No evaluation of this step.

Instructor shall define grades for each point range earned upon completion of each performance-evaluated task.

Performance Standards

The minimum number of satisfactory performances required prior to final evaluation is _____.

Instructor shall identify by * those steps considered critical. If step is missed or minimum competency is not met, the evaluated procedure fails and must be repeated.

Performance Criteria	*	Self	Peer	Instructor	Comments
1. Washes hands and dons gloves.					
2. Places a new sheath over the probe of the digital thermometer.					
3. Turns the thermometer on. When the display indicates that it is ready, instructs patient to raise their tongue to the roof of their mouth and gently places the tip under the patient's tongue.					
4. Instructs the patient to close his or her lips over the thermometer and to refrain from talking or removing it from the mouth.					
5. Leaves the thermometer in place until the display indicates a final reading; removes thermometer from the patient's mouth.					
6. Records the reading in the patient record.					
7. Turns the thermometer off, removes the sheath, and disinfects the thermometer as recommended by the manufacturer.					
Additional Comments					

Total number of points possible _____

Total number of points received _____

Grade _____ Instructor's initials _____ Date _____

COMPETENCY 9-4 TAKING A PATIENT'S PULSE

Performance Objective

By following a routine procedure that meets stated protocols, the student will be able to take a patient's pulse.

Evaluation and Grading Criteria

3   Student competently met the stated criteria without assistance.

2   Student required assistance in order to meet the stated criteria.

1   Student showed uncertainty when performing the stated criteria.

0   Student was not prepared and needs to repeat the step.

N/A   No evaluation of this step.

Instructor shall define grades for each point range earned upon completion of each performance-evaluated task.

Performance Standards

The minimum number of satisfactory performances required prior to final evaluation is _____.

Instructor shall identify by * those steps considered critical. If step is missed or minimum competency is not met, the evaluated procedure fails and must be repeated.

Performance Criteria	*	Self	Peer	Instructor	Comments
1. Patient is seated in an upright position.					
2. Extends the patient's arm and positions it on the armrest of the chair, making sure the arm is at or below the heart level.					
3. Places the tips of index and middle fingers on the patient's radial artery.					
4. Feels for the patient's pulse before beginning to count.					
5. Counts the beats for 30 seconds then multiplies by 2 to compute the rate for a 1-minute reading.					
6. Records the rate, along with any distinct changes in the rhythm in the patient record.					
Additional Comments					

Total number of points possible _____

Total number of points received _____

Grade _____ *Instructor's initials* _____ *Date* _____

Performance Objective

By following a routine procedure that meets stated protocols, the student will be able to measure a patient's respiration.

Evaluation and Grading Criteria

3	Student competently met the stated criteria without assistance.
2	Student required assistance in order to meet the stated criteria.
1	Student showed uncertainty when performing the stated criteria.
0	Student was not prepared and needs to repeat the step.
N/A	No evaluation of this step.

Instructor shall define grades for each point range earned upon completion of each performance-evaluated task.

Performance Standards

The minimum number of satisfactory performances required prior to final evaluation is _____.

Instructor shall identify by * those steps considered critical. If step is missed or minimum competency is not met, the evaluated procedure fails and must be repeated.

Performance Criteria	*	Self	Peer	Instructor	Comments
1. Patient remains seated and assistant maintains the position used while taking the pulse.					
2. Counts the rise and fall of the patient's chest for 30 seconds then multiplies by 2 to compute the rate for a 1-minute reading.					
3. Enters the rate, rhythm, and depth in the patient's record.					
Additional Comments					

Total number of points possible _____

Total number of points received _____

Grade _____ *Instructor's initials* _____ *Date* _____

COMPETENCY 9-6 TAKING A PATIENT'S BLOOD PRESSURE

Performance Objective

By following a routine procedure that meets stated protocols, the student will be able to take a patient's blood pressure.

Evaluation and Grading Criteria

3   Student competently met the stated criteria without assistance.

2   Student required assistance in order to meet the stated criteria.

1   Student showed uncertainty when performing the stated criteria.

0   Student was not prepared and needs to repeat the step.

N/A   No evaluation of this step.

Instructor shall define grades for each point range earned upon completion of each performance-evaluated task.

Performance Standards

The minimum number of satisfactory performances required prior to final evaluation is _____.

Instructor shall identify by * those steps considered critical. If step is missed or minimum competency is not met, the evaluated procedure fails and must be repeated.

Performance Criteria	*	Self	Peer	Instructor	Comments
1. Patient seated in an upright positon with his or her arm extended at heart level and supported on the chair's armrest.					
2. If possible, rolls up the patient's sleeve.					
For a patient's First Reading					
1. Establishes a basis to determine how high to inflate the cuff by palpating the brachial artery and detecting the patient's pulse.					
2. Takes the patient's brachial pulse for 30 seconds then multiplies by 2 for a 1-minute reading. Adds 40 mm Hg to the reading and provides for inflation level.					
Cuff Application					
1. Expels any air from the cuff by opening the valve and pressing gently on the cuff.					
2. Places the blood pressure cuff around the patient's arm approximately 1 inch above the antecubital space, making sure to center the arrow over the brachial artery.					
3. Tightens the cuff, using the Velcro closure to hold it in place.					
4. Places the earpieces of the stethoscope into ears so that they are facing toward the front.					
5. Places the stethoscope disc over the site of the brachial artery, using slight pressure with the fingers.					

63

Performance Criteria	*	Self	Peer	Instructor	Comments
6. Grasps the rubber bulb with the other hand, locking the valve. Inflates the cuff to the inflation reading.					
7. Slowly releases the valve and listens through the stethoscope.					
8. Identifies the first distinct thumping sound as the cuff deflates. This is the systolic reading.					
9. Slowly continues to release the air from the cuff until the last sound is heard. This is the diastolic reading.					
10. Records the reading, indicating which arm was used.					
11. Disinfects the stethoscope earpieces and diaphragm as recommended by the manufacturer.					
12. Returns the setup to its proper place.					
Additional Comments					

Total number of points possible _____

Total number of points received _____

Grade _____ *Instructor's initials* _____ *Date* _____

10 Medical Emergencies in the Dental Office

TRUE/FALSE

_____ 1. The best way to help prevent a potential medical emergency is to have a complete and updated medical history.

_____ 2. The standard of care for an emergency procedure requires the dental assistant to be competent in CPR and administer lifesaving drugs.

_____ 3. A list of emergency phone numbers should be noted in the patient record.

_____ 4. Oxygen is the most frequently used drug in a medical emergency.

_____ 5. The diagnosis of a medical emergency is the responsibility of everyone on the dental team.

_____ 6. The front desk staff member would be most likely to call for emergency service and then remain on the phone.

_____ 7. An EpiPen can be used for anaphylactic shock.

_____ 8. A patient with a history of angina would commonly carry albuterol for chest pain.

_____ 9. A "sign" is what you observe in the patient experiencing an emergency.

_____ 10. In most areas, the emergency medical service (EMS) can be reached at 919.

MATCHING

_____ 11. Sudden coughing, clutching their throat

_____ 12. Localized itching

_____ 13. Abnormal increase in blood glucose

_____ 14. Wheezing with narrowing airway

_____ 15. Patient placed in upright position too quickly

_____ 16. Severe chest pain

_____ 17. Rapid, shallow breathing

_____ 18. Interruption of blood flow to the brain

_____ 19. Commonly known as "fainting"

_____ 20. Neurologic disorder

_____ 21. Heart attack

A. Syncope

B. Postural hypotension

C. Hyperventilation

D. Airway obstruction

E. Asthma

F. Allergic reaction

G. Angina

H. Myocardial infarction

I. Hyperglycemia

J. Cerebrovascular accident

K. Seizure

SHORT ANSWER

22. List the commonly assigned responsibilities of the following members of the dental team in an emergency situation:

a. Business assistant _____

_____

b. Clinical assistant and/or dental hygienist

_____

_____

c. Dentist (clinical assistant or dental hygienist)

_____

_____

d. Other team members _____

_____

_____

23. Describe the difference between a "symptom" and a "sign".

COMPETENCY 10-1 PERFORMING CARDIOPULMONARY RESUSCITATION (CPR) (ONE PERSON)

Performance Objective

By following a routine procedure that meets stated protocols, the student will be able to perform cardiopulmonary resuscitation on one person.

Evaluation and Grading Criteria

3   Student competently met the stated criteria without assistance.

2   Student required assistance in order to meet the stated criteria.

1   Student showed uncertainty when performing the stated criteria.

0   Student was not prepared and needs to repeat the step.

N/A   No evaluation of this step.

Instructor shall define grades for each point range earned upon completion of each performance-evaluated task.

Performance Standards

The minimum number of satisfactory performances required prior to final evaluation is _____.

Instructor shall identify by * those steps considered critical. If step is missed or minimum competency is not met, the evaluated procedure fails and must be repeated.

Performance Criteria	*	Self	Peer	Instructor	Comments
Determine Unresponsiveness Approaches the victim and checks for signs of circulation, such as normal breathing, coughing, or movement in response to stimulation. Pinches or taps the victim and asks, "Are you OK?"					
Initiate Assistance If there is no response, calls for assistance and asks someone to call 911; obtains an AED/defibrillator if available. If alone and patient is an adult, phones 911 first and then begins compressions. If the patient is a child, gives 2 minutes of compressions first, then calls 911.					
Initiate Compressions 1. Kneels at the victim's side, opposite the chest. Moves fingers up the ribs to the point where the sternum and the ribs join. Fits middle finger into the area and places index finger next to it across the sternum.					
2. Places heel of the hand on the chest midline over the sternum, just above index finger. Places other hand on top of first hand and lifts fingers upward off the chest.					
3. Has shoulders directly over the victim's sternum, compressed downward, and keeps arms straight.					

67

Performance Criteria	*	Self	Peer	Instructor	Comments
4. Provides 30 chest compressions at a rate of 100/ minute with adequate depth. Specific techniques remembered during compression are: • Push hard and fast. • Allow complete chest recoil after each compression. • Minimize interruptions in compressions. • Avoid excessive ventilation. • If multiple rescuers are available, rotate task of compressions every 2 minutes.					
5. For adults and children older than 8 years, compresses the chest a depth of at least 2 inches.					
6. For infants and children under 8, compresses the chest a depth of 1½ inches.					
Airway and Ventilation 1. Opening the airway (followed by rescue breaths) should be completed only if there are two rescuers and one of the rescuers is trained in CPR.					
2. Once chest compressions are started, a trained rescuer should deliver rescue breaths by mouth-to-mouth or bag-mask to provide oxygenation and ventilation, as follows: • Deliver each rescue breath over 1 second. • Give a sufficient tidal volume to produce visible chest rise. • Use a compression-to-ventilation ratio of 30 chest compressions to 2 ventilations.					
3. Repeats ongoing cycles of CPR until EMS arrives, the person starts breathing, someone comes with an AED, or another trained rescuer takes over.					
Additional Comments					

Total number of points possible _____

Total number of points received _____

Grade _____ Instructor's initials _____ Date _____

Performance Objective

By following a routine procedure that meets stated protocols, the student will demonstrate the proper technique for operating an automated external defibrillator in an emergency situation.

Evaluation and Grading Criteria

3	Student competently met the stated criteria without assistance.
2	Student required assistance in order to meet the stated criteria.
1	Student showed uncertainty when performing the stated criteria.
0	Student was not prepared and needs to repeat the step.
N/A	No evaluation of this step.

Instructor shall define grades for each point range earned on completion of each performance-evaluated task.

Performance Standards

The minimum number of satisfactory performances required before final evaluation is _____.

Instructor shall identify by * those steps considered critical. If a step is missed or minimum competency is not met, the evaluated procedure fails and must be repeated.

Performance Criteria	*	Self	Peer	Instructor	Comments
1. Verified the absence of breathing and pulse.					
2. Began CPR.					
3. Positioned the defibrillator machine on the left side of the patient's head.					
4. Turned the power on.					
5. Attached the electrode lines to the paddles.					
6. Attached the paddles to the patient. Positioned one paddle at the left sternal border and the second on the right side above the nipple area.					
7. Stopped CPR and cleared the patient.					
8. Pressed the "analyze" button.					
9. If the machine advised shock, delivered a shock.					

Performance Criteria	*	Self	Peer	Instructor	Comments
10. Reanalyzed the cardiac rhythm. Completed three intervals and then reassessed.					
11. Documented procedure in patient record.					
Additional Comments					

Total number of points earned _____

Grade _____ Instructor's initials _____

COMPETENCY 10-3 RESPONDING TO A PATIENT WITH AN OBSTRUCTED AIRWAY

Performance Objective

By following a routine procedure that meets stated protocols, the student will be able to respond to a patient with an obstructed airway.

Evaluation and Grading Criteria

3   Student competently met the stated criteria without assistance.

2   Student required assistance in order to meet the stated criteria.

1   Student showed uncertainty when performing the stated criteria.

0   Student was not prepared and needs to repeat the step.

N/A   No evaluation of this step.

Instructor shall define grades for each point range earned upon completion of each performance-evaluated task.

Performance Standards

The minimum number of satisfactory performances required prior to final evaluation is _____.

Instructor shall identify by ∗ those steps considered critical. If step is missed or minimum competency is not met, the evaluated procedure fails and must be repeated.

Performance Criteria	∗	Self	Peer	Instructor	Comments
Care of the Patient					
1. If a patient cannot speak, cough, or breathe, the airway is completely blocked. Immediately calls for assistance and begins administering the Heimlich maneuver.					
2. Makes a fist with one hand and places thumb side of hand against the patient's abdomen, just above the navel and below the xiphoid process of the sternum.					
3. Grasps the fist with the other hand and forcefully thrusts both hands into the abdomen, using an inward and upward motion.					
4. Repeats the thrusts until the object is expelled.					

71

Performance Criteria	*	Self	Peer	Instructor	Comments
Responding to the Conscious Seated Patient					
1. Positions patient either standing or on flat surface before administering the Heimlich maneuver.					
2. Places the heel of one hand at the patient's abdomen above the navel and well below the xiphoid process.					
3. Places the other hand directly over the first hand. Administers a firm, quick, upward thrust into the patient's diaphragm.					
4. Repeats this maneuver 6–10 times as needed until the object is dislodged or until advanced emergency assistance arrives.					
Additional Comments					

Total number of points possible _____

Total number of points received _____

Grade _____ *Instructor's initials* _____ *Date* _____

Performance Objective

By following a routine procedure that meets stated protocols, the student will be able to respond to an unconscious patient.

Evaluation and Grading Criteria

3	Student competently met the stated criteria without assistance.
2	Student required assistance in order to meet the stated criteria.
1	Student showed uncertainty when performing the stated criteria.
0	Student was not prepared and needs to repeat the step.
N/A	No evaluation of this step.

Instructor shall define grades for each point range earned upon completion of each performance-evaluated task.

Performance Standards

The minimum number of satisfactory performances required prior to final evaluation is _____.

Instructor shall identify by ∗ those steps considered critical. If step is missed or minimum competency is not met, the evaluated procedure fails and must be repeated.

Performance Criteria	∗	Self	Peer	Instructor	Comments
Syncope (Fainting)					
1. Places the patient in a subsupine position with his or her head lower than the feet.					
2. Loosens any binding clothes on the patient.					
3. Has an ammonia inhalant ready to administer by waving it under the patient's nose several times.					
4. Has oxygen ready to administer.					
5. Calls for emergency assistance (911).					
6. Monitors and records patient's vital signs.					
Postural Hypotension					
1. Places the patient in a subsupine position with his or her head lower than the feet.					
2. Establishes an airway.					
3. Slowly moves the patient into an upright position.					
4. If the patient does not respond immediately, calls for emergency assistance (911).					
5. Monitors and records vital signs.					
Additional Comments					

Total number of points possible _____

Total number of points received _____

Grade _____ *Instructor's initials* _____ *Date* _____

73

Performance Objective

By following a routine procedure that meets stated protocols, the student will be able to respond to a patient with breathing difficulty.

Evaluation and Grading Criteria

3   Student competently met the stated criteria without assistance.

2   Student required assistance in order to meet the stated criteria.

1   Student showed uncertainty when performing the stated criteria.

0   Student was not prepared and needs to repeat the step.

N/A   No evaluation of this step.

Instructor shall define grades for each point range earned upon completion of each performance-evaluated task.

Performance Standards

The minimum number of satisfactory performances required prior to final evaluation is _____.

Instructor shall identify by * those steps considered critical. If step is missed or minimum competency is not met, the evaluated procedure fails and must be repeated.

Performance Criteria	*	Self	Peer	Instructor	Comments
Hyperventilation 1. Places the patient in a comfortable position.					
2. Uses a quiet tone of voice to calm and reassure the patient.					
3. Instructs the patient to breathe into his or her cupped hands.					
Asthma Attack 1. Calls for assistance.					
2. Positions the patient as comfortable as possible (upright is best).					
3. Has patient self-medicate with inhaler.					
4. Administers oxygen as needed.					
Additional Comments					

Total number of points possible _____

Total number of points received _____

Grade _____ *Instructor's initials* _____ *Date* _____

COMPETENCY 10-6 RESPONDING TO THE PATIENT EXPERIENCING A SEIZURE

Performance Objective

By following a routine procedure that meets stated protocols, the student will be able to respond to a patient experiencing a convulsive seizure.

Evaluation and Grading Criteria

3   Student competently met the stated criteria without assistance.

2   Student required assistance in order to meet the stated criteria.

1   Student showed uncertainty when performing the stated criteria.

0   Student was not prepared and needs to repeat the step.

N/A   No evaluation of this step.

Instructor shall define grades for each point range earned upon completion of each performance-evaluated task.

Performance Standards

The minimum number of satisfactory performances required prior to final evaluation is _____.

Instructor shall identify by ∗ those steps considered critical. If step is missed or minimum competency is not met, the evaluated procedure fails and must be repeated.

Performance Criteria	∗	Self	Peer	Instructor	Comments
Generalized Seizure					
1. Calls for emergency assistance (911).					
2. If seizure occurs while the patient is in the dental chair, quickly removes all materials from the mouth and places the patient in a supine position.					
3. Protects the patient from self-injury during convulsions.					
4. Prepares to use anticonvulsant (diazepam) from the drug kit.					
5. Initiates basic life support (CPR) if needed.					
6. Monitors and records vital signs.					
Partial Seizure					
1. Calls for emergency assistance (911).					
2. Prevents injury to patient.					
3. Monitors and records vital signs.					
4. Refers patient for medical consultation.					
Additional Comments					

Total number of points possible _____

Total number of points received _____

Grade _____ *Instructor's initials* _____ *Date* _____

77

COMPETENCY 10-7 RESPONDING TO THE PATIENT EXPERIENCING A DIABETIC EMERGENCY

Performance Objective

By following a routine procedure that meets stated protocols, the student will be able to respond to a patient experiencing a diabetic emergency.

Evaluation and Grading Criteria

3   Student competently met the stated criteria without assistance.

2   Student required assistance in order to meet the stated criteria.

1   Student showed uncertainty when performing the stated criteria.

0   Student was not prepared and needs to repeat the step.

N/A   No evaluation of this step.

Instructor shall define grades for each point range earned upon completion of each performance-evaluated task.

Performance Standards

The minimum number of satisfactory performances required prior to final evaluation is _____.

Instructor shall identify by * those steps considered critical. If step is missed or minimum competency is not met, the evaluated procedure fails and must be repeated.

Performance Criteria	*	Self	Peer	Instructor	Comments
Hyperglycemia 1. Calls for emergency assistance (911).					
2. If the patient is conscious, asks when he or she last ate, whether the patient has taken insulin, and whether he or she brought insulin with him or her to the dental appointment.					
3. Retrieves the patient's insulin if it is available. Has the patient self-administer the insulin if able.					
4. Provides basic life support (CPR) if the patient becomes unconscious.					
5. Monitors and records vital signs.					
Hypoglycemia 1. Calls for emergency assistance (911).					
2. If patient is conscious, asks when he or she last ate, whether the patient has taken insulin, and whether he or she brought insulin with him or her to the dental appointment.					
3. If the patient is conscious, gives a concentrated form of carbohydrate, such as a sugar packet, cake icing, or concentrated orange juice.					

Performance Criteria	*	Self	Peer	Instructor	Comments
4. Provides basic life support (CPR) if the patient becomes unconscious.					
5. Monitors and records vital signs.					
Additional Comments					

Total number of points possible _____

Total number of points received _____

Grade _____ *Instructor's initials* _____ *Date* _____

Performance Objective

By following a routine procedure that meets stated protocols, the student will be able to respond to a patient with chest pain.

Evaluation and Grading Criteria

3   Student competently met the stated criteria without assistance.

2   Student required assistance in order to meet the stated criteria.

1   Student showed uncertainty when performing the stated criteria.

0   Student was not prepared and needs to repeat the step.

N/A   No evaluation of this step.

Instructor shall define grades for each point range earned upon completion of each performance-evaluated task.

Performance Standards

The minimum number of satisfactory performances required prior to final evaluation is _____.

Instructor shall identify by * those steps considered critical. If step is missed or minimum competency is not met, the evaluated procedure fails and must be repeated.

Performance Criteria	*	Self	Peer	Instructor	Comments
Angina Attack 1. Calls for emergency assistance (911).					
2. Positions the patient upright.					
3. If possible, have the patient self-medicate with nitroglycerin supply (tablets, spray, or topical cream).					
4. Administers oxygen.					
5. Monitors and records vital signs.					
Acute Myocardial Infarction (Heart Attack) 1. Calls for emergency assistance (911).					
2. Have the patient positioned comfortably.					
3. Initiates basic life support (CPR) if the patient becomes unconscious.					
4. If the patient has prescribed nitroglycerin, administer that or obtain from the emergency kit.					
5. If the person is not allergic to aspirin and is not taking blood thinners, give 2 to 4 chewable baby aspirins (81 mg each) or one adult aspirin (325 mg) with a small amount of water.					

81

Performance Criteria	*	Self	Peer	Instructor	Comments
6. Administers oxygen.					
7. Monitors and records vital signs.					
Additional Comments					

Total number of points possible _____

Total number of points received _____

Grade _____ *Instructor's initials* _____ *Date* _____

Performance Objective

By following a routine procedure that meets stated protocols, the student will be able to respond to a patient experiencing a stroke.

Evaluation and Grading Criteria

3	Student competently met the stated criteria without assistance.
2	Student required assistance in order to meet the stated criteria.
1	Student showed uncertainty when performing the stated criteria.
0	Student was not prepared and needs to repeat the step.
N/A	No evaluation of this step.

Instructor shall define grades for each point range earned upon completion of each performance-evaluated task.

Performance Standards

The minimum number of satisfactory performances required prior to final evaluation is _____.

Instructor shall identify by * those steps considered critical. If step is missed or minimum competency is not met, the evaluated procedure fails and must be repeated.

Performance Criteria	*	Self	Peer	Instructor	Comments
1. Calls for emergency assistance (911).					
2. Initiates basic life support (CPR) if the patient becomes unconscious.					
3. Monitors and records vital signs.					
Additional Comments					

Total number of points possible _____

Total number of points received _____

Grade _____ *Instructor's initials* _____ *Date* _____

COMPETENCY 10-10 RESPONDING TO THE PATIENT EXPERIENCING AN ALLERGIC REACTION

Performance Objective

By following a routine procedure that meets stated protocols, the student will be able to respond to a patient experiencing an allergic reaction.

Evaluation and Grading Criteria

3   Student competently met the stated criteria without assistance.

2   Student required assistance in order to meet the stated criteria.

1   Student showed uncertainty when performing the stated criteria.

0   Student was not prepared and needs to repeat the step.

N/A   No evaluation of this step.

Instructor shall define grades for each point range earned upon completion of each performance-evaluated task.

Performance Standards

The minimum number of satisfactory performances required prior to final evaluation is _____.

Instructor shall identify by * those steps considered critical. If step is missed or minimum competency is not met, the evaluated procedure fails and must be repeated.

Performance Criteria	*	Self	Peer	Instructor	Comments
Localized Rash					
1. Observes patient for advanced signs or symptoms.					
2. Prepares an EpiPen® for administration.					
3. Is prepared to administer basic life support (CPR) if necessary.					
4. Refers the patient for medical consultation.					
Anaphylaxis					
1. Calls for emergency assistance (911).					
2. Places the patient in a supine position.					
3. Starts basic life support (CPR) if patient becomes unconscious.					
4. Prepares to assist in the administration of the EpiPen®.					
5. Administers oxygen.					
6. Monitors and records vital signs.					
Additional Comments					

Total number of points possible _____

Total number of points received _____

Grade _____ *Instructor's initials* _____ *Date* _____

11 Delivering Dental Care

TRUE/FALSE

_____ 1. The dental treatment area is also referred to as the dental ambulatory center.

_____ 2. A standard routine procedure must be followed when admitting and positioning the patient and dental team.

_____ 3. The patient's personal items should be handed to the front desk staff for safekeeping while the patient is being seen.

_____ 4. In a subsupine position, the patient's head is actually lower than their feet.

_____ 5. The science that seeks to adapt working conditions to suit workers is ergonomics.

_____ 6. For correct operator positioning, the operator should be positioned approximately 4–5 inches higher than the assistant.

_____ 7. A painful condition associated with continued flexion and extension of the wrist is carpal tunnel syndrome.

_____ 8. An instrument is exchanged from the assistant to the dentist in the transfer zone.

_____ 9. At the beginning of a procedure, the mouth mirror and air-water syringe are transferred to the operator to examine the area to be treated.

_____ 10. Throughout a procedure for a right-handed operator, the dental assistant uses the left hand to transfer instruments while holding the oral evacuation system in the right hand.

MATCHING

Match the following dental treatment equipment to its description:

_____ 11. Dental chair

_____ 12. Curing light

_____ 13. Dental unit

_____ 14. Operator's stool

_____ 15. Oral evacuation

_____ 16. Operating light

_____ 17. Assistant's stool

_____ 18. Air-water syringe

_____ 19. Amalgamator

A. Illuminates the oral cavity

B. Designed to support the patient comfortably

C. Provides stability, mobility, and comfort for the assistant

D. Provides the electricity and air to equipment

E. Used to rinse or dry areas of the mouth

F. Supports the operator for long periods of time

G. Triturates encapsulated dental materials

H. Removes fluids and debris from the mouth

I. Activates the polymerization of resins and composites

SHORT ANSWER

20. Describe the four goals that the dental assistant and dentist should work together to accomplish.

21. List the specific criteria for proper positioning of the seated operator.

22. List the specific criteria for proper positioning of the seated dental assistant.

23. Name the three types of operator grasps commonly used when receiving an instrument.

LABELING

24. Using the diagram below, label each zone and describe what should be in each of those areas.

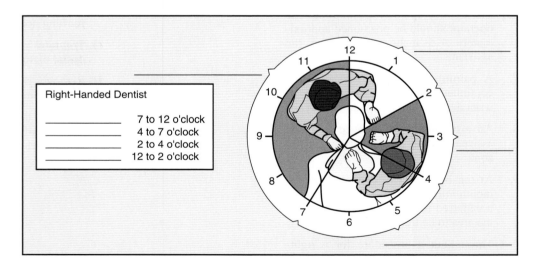

Right-Handed Dentist

_____	7 to 12 o'clock
_____	4 to 7 o'clock
_____	2 to 4 o'clock
_____	12 to 2 o'clock

COMPETENCY 11-1 ADMITTING AND SEATING THE PATIENT

Performance Objective

By following a routine procedure that meets stated protocols, the student will be able to properly admit and seat the patient.

Evaluation and Grading Criteria

3   Student competently met the stated criteria without assistance.

2   Student required assistance in order to meet the stated criteria.

1   Student showed uncertainty when performing the stated criteria.

0   Student was not prepared and needs to repeat the step.

N/A   No evaluation of this step.

Instructor shall define grades for each point range earned upon completion of each performance-evaluated task.

Performance Standards

The minimum number of satisfactory performances required prior to final evaluation is _____.

Instructor shall identify by ∗ those steps considered critical. If step is missed or minimum competency is not met, the evaluated procedure fails and must be repeated.

Performance Criteria	∗	Self	Peer	Instructor	Comments
1. Ensured that the treatment room is properly cleaned and prepared, with the chair properly positioned and the patient's path clear.					
2. Pleasantly greets the patient in the reception area by name. Introduces self and requests that the patient follow him or her to the treatment area.					
3. Places the patient's personal items in a safe place away from the procedure but within eye view for patient.					
4. Initiates conversation with the patient.					
5. Asks the patient if he or she has any questions about treatment for the day. If the assistant does not know the answer, he or she says so and offers to discuss this with the dentist.					
6. Seats patient properly in dental chair by having him or her sit on the side of the chair and swing his or her legs onto the base of the chair.					
7. Positions the chair arm.					
8. Places the disposable patient napkin over the patient's chest and clasps the corners using a napkin chain.					
9. Informs the patient before adjusting the chair. Makes the adjustments slowly until the patient and chair are in the proper position for the planned procedure.					

Performance Criteria	*	Self	Peer	Instructor	Comments
10. Positions the operating light over the patient's chest and turns it on.					
11. All treatment room preparations are organized and set out.					
Additional Comments					

Total number of points possible _____

Total number of points received _____

Grade _____ *Instructor's initials* _____ *Date* _____

COMPETENCY 11-2 TRANSFERRING INSTRUMENTS USING THE SINGLE-HANDED TECHNIQUE

Performance Objective

By following a routine procedure that meets stated protocols, the student will be able to properly transfer instruments using the single-handed technique.

Evaluation and Grading Criteria

3   Student competently met the stated criteria without assistance.

2   Student required assistance in order to meet the stated criteria.

1   Student showed uncertainty when performing the stated criteria.

0   Student was not prepared and needs to repeat the step.

N/A   No evaluation of this step.

Instructor shall define grades for each point range earned upon completion of each performance-evaluated task.

Performance Standards

The minimum number of satisfactory performances required prior to final evaluation is _____.

Instructor shall identify by ∗ those steps considered critical. If step is missed or minimum competency is not met, the evaluated procedure fails and must be repeated.

Performance Criteria	∗	Self	Peer	Instructor	Comments
1. Personal protective equipment placed according to procedure.					
2. Retrieves the instrument from the tray setup using the thumb, index finger, and middle finger of left hand.					
3. Grasps the instrument at the end of the handle or opposite the working end.					
4. Transfers the instrument from the tray into the transfer zone, ensuring that the instrument is parallel to the instrument in the dentist's hand and below the patients chin.					
5. Using the last two fingers of the left hand, retrieves the used instrument from the dentist, tucking the instrument in toward the palm.					
6. Positions the new instrument firmly in the dentist's fingers.					
7. Returns the used instrument to its proper position on the tray.					
8. Maintains safety throughout the transfer.					
Additional Comments					

Total number of points possible _____

Total number of points received _____

Grade _____ *Instructor's initials* _____ *Date* _____

     Chapter **11**   **Delivering Dental Care**

COMPETENCY 11-3 TRANSFERRING INSTRUMENTS USING THE TWO-HANDED TECHNIQUE

Performance Objective

By following a routine procedure that meets stated protocols, the student will be able to properly transfer instruments using a two-handed technique.

Evaluation and Grading Criteria

3   Student competently met the stated criteria without assistance.

2   Student required assistance in order to meet the stated criteria.

1   Student showed uncertainty when performing the stated criteria.

0   Student was not prepared and needs to repeat the step.

N/A   No evaluation of this step.

Instructor shall define grades for each point range earned upon completion of each performance-evaluated task.

Performance Standards

The minimum number of satisfactory performances required prior to final evaluation is _____.

Instructor shall identify by ∗ those steps considered critical. If step is missed or minimum competency is not met, the evaluated procedure fails and must be repeated.

Performance Criteria	∗	Self	Peer	Instructor	Comments
1. Uses right hand to grasp instrument from the tray setup closer to the working end with thumb and first two fingers.					
2. With left hand, retrieves the used instrument from dentist, using the reverse palm grasp to hold the instrument before placing it back on tray.					
3. Delivers the new instrument to the dentist so that it is oriented with the working end in the appropriate position.					
4. Returns the used instrument to its proper position on the tray.					
Additional Comments					

Total number of points possible _____

Total number of points received _____

Grade _____ *Instructor's initials* _____ *Date* _____

12 Instruments, Handpieces, and Accessories

TRUE/FALSE

_____ 1. Examination instruments are used to remove decay and prepare tooth structure for its restoration.

_____ 2. Each hand instrument is made up of three parts: the handle, shank, and working end.

_____ 3. For a right-handed operator, instruments are sequenced on a tray specifically to be used from right to left.

_____ 4. A rotary instrument is useless unless it is attached to a dental handpiece.

_____ 5. Disposable prophy angles should be sterilized after use.

_____ 6. A long straight-shank portion of the bur will fit into the straight attachment of the low-speed handpiece.

_____ 7. Torque is the turning power of the instrument when pressure is applied.

_____ 8. The high-speed handpiece is equipped with a fiberoptic light.

_____ 9. Finishing burs are similar to carbide burs except the blades are not as sharp and are farther apart.

_____ 10. A mandrel is attached to the high-speed handpiece when using polishing discs.

MATCHING

_____ 11. Mouth mirror

_____ 12. Spoon excavator

_____ 13. Amalgam carrier

_____ 14. Burnisher

_____ 15. Amalgam condenser

_____ 16. Hatchet

_____ 17. Cotton pliers

_____ 18. Hollenback

_____ 19. Discoid/cleoid

_____ 20. Explorer

A. Used to carry, place, and remove items in the mouth

B. Used to examine healthy and diseased tooth structure

C. Carves amalgam on the occlusal surface

D. Prepares the walls and floors of a tooth preparation

E. Removes soft dentin, debris, and decay

F. Carves amalgam at proximal surfaces

G. Carries amalgam to the prepared tooth

H. Smooths amalgam on the occlusal surface

I. Improves view, reflects light, retracts, and protects tissue carver

J. Packs amalgam into the tooth preparation

SHORT ANSWER

21. List the four categories of dental hand instruments and describe their functions.

22. Fill in the name, number series, and use of each bur shape below.

A.

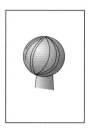

(From Finkbeiner BL, Johnson CS: *Mosby's comprehensive dental assisting*, St Louis, 1995, Mosby.)

Name: _____

Number series: _____

Use: _____

B.

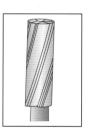

(From Finkbeiner BL, Johnson CS: *Mosby's comprehensive dental assisting*, St Louis, 1995, Mosby.)

Name: _____

Number series: _____

Use: _____

C.

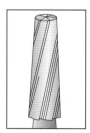

(From Finkbeiner BL, Johnson CS: *Mosby's comprehensive dental assisting*, St Louis, 1995, Mosby.)

Name: _____

Number series: _____

Use: _____

D.

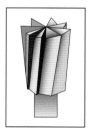

(From Baum L, Phillips RW, Lund MR: *Textbook of operative dentistry*, ed 3, Philadelphia, 1995, Saunders.)

Name: _____

Number series: _____

Use: _____

E.

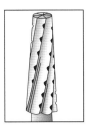

(From Finkbeiner BL, Johnson CS: *Mosby's comprehensive dental assisting*, St Louis, 1995, Mosby.)

Name: _____

Number series: _____

Use: _____

F.

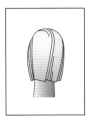

(From Finkbeiner BL, Johnson CS: *Mosby's comprehensive dental assisting*, St Louis, 1995, Mosby.)

Name: _____

Number series: _____

Use: _____

Performance Objective

By following a routine procedure that meets stated protocols, the student will be able to identify the examination instruments.

Evaluation and Grading Criteria

3	Student competently met the stated criteria without assistance.
2	Student required assistance in order to meet the stated criteria.
1	Student showed uncertainty when performing the stated criteria.
0	Student was not prepared and needs to repeat the step.
N/A	No evaluation of this step.

Instructor shall define grades for each point range earned upon completion of each performance-evaluated task.

Performance Standards

The minimum number of satisfactory performances required prior to final evaluation is _____.

Instructor shall identify by ∗ those steps considered critical. If step is missed or minimum competency is not met, the evaluated procedure fails and must be repeated.

Performance Criteria	∗	Self	Peer	Instructor	Comments
1. Writes the general classification of the instrument.					
2. Writes the complete name of each instrument or item and spells it correctly.					
3. Identifies its use.					
Additional Comments					

Total number of points possible _____

Total number of points received _____

Grade _____ Instructor's initials _____ Date _____

COMPETENCY 12-2 IDENTIFYING HAND (MANUAL) CUTTING INSTRUMENTS

Performance Objective

By following a routine procedure that meets stated protocols, the student will be able to identify the hand (manual) cutting instruments.

Evaluation and Grading Criteria

3   Student competently met the stated criteria without assistance.

2   Student required assistance in order to meet the stated criteria.

1   Student showed uncertainty when performing the stated criteria.

0   Student was not prepared and needs to repeat the step.

N/A   No evaluation of this step.

Instructor shall define grades for each point range earned upon completion of each performance-evaluated task.

Performance Standards

The minimum number of satisfactory performances required prior to final evaluation is _____.

Instructor shall identify by ∗ those steps considered critical. If step is missed or minimum competency is not met, the evaluated procedure fails and must be repeated.

Performance Criteria	∗	Self	Peer	Instructor	Comments
1. Writes the general classification of the instrument.					
2. Writes the complete name of each instrument or item and spells it correctly.					
3. Identifies its use.					
Additional Comments					

Total number of points possible _____

Total number of points received _____

Grade _____ Instructor's initials _____ Date _____

101

Performance Objective

By following a routine procedure that meets stated protocols, the student will be able to identify the restorative instruments.

Evaluation and Grading Criteria

3   Student competently met the stated criteria without assistance.

2   Student required assistance in order to meet the stated criteria.

1   Student showed uncertainty when performing the stated criteria.

0   Student was not prepared and needs to repeat the step.

N/A   No evaluation of this step.

Instructor shall define grades for each point range earned upon completion of each performance-evaluated task.

Performance Standards

The minimum number of satisfactory performances required prior to final evaluation is _____.

Instructor shall identify by ∗ those steps considered critical. If step is missed or minimum competency is not met, the evaluated procedure fails and must be repeated.

Performance Criteria	∗	Self	Peer	Instructor	Comments
1. Writes the general classification of the instrument.					
2. Writes the complete name of each instrument or item and spells it correctly.					
3. Identifies its use.					
Additional Comments					

Total number of points possible _____

Total number of points received _____

Grade _____ Instructor's initials _____ Date _____

COMPETENCY 12-4 IDENTIFYING ACCESSORY INSTRUMENTS AND ITEMS

Performance Objective

By following a routine procedure that meets stated protocols, the student will be able to identify the accessory instruments and items.

Evaluation and Grading Criteria

3   Student competently met the stated criteria without assistance.

2   Student required assistance in order to meet the stated criteria.

1   Student showed uncertainty when performing the stated criteria.

0   Student was not prepared and needs to repeat the step.

N/A   No evaluation of this step.

Instructor shall define grades for each point range earned upon completion of each performance-evaluated task.

Performance Standards

The minimum number of satisfactory performances required prior to final evaluation is _____.

Instructor shall identify by * those steps considered critical. If step is missed or minimum competency is not met, the evaluated procedure fails and must be repeated.

Performance Criteria	*	Self	Peer	Instructor	Comments
1. Writes the general classification of the instrument.					
2. Writes the complete name of each instrument or item and spells it correctly.					
3. Identifies its use.					
Additional Comments					

Total number of points possible _____

Total number of points received _____

Grade _____ *Instructor's initials* _____ *Date* _____

105

COMPETENCY 12-5 IDENTIFYING AND ATTACHING THE DENTAL HANDPIECE

Performance Objective

By following a routine procedure that meets stated protocols, the student will be able to identify and attach a dental handpiece.

Evaluation and Grading Criteria

3   Student competently met the stated criteria without assistance.

2   Student required assistance in order to meet the stated criteria.

1   Student showed uncertainty when performing the stated criteria.

0   Student was not prepared and needs to repeat the step.

N/A   No evaluation of this step.

Instructor shall define grades for each point range earned upon completion of each performance-evaluated task.

Performance Standards

The minimum number of satisfactory performances required prior to final evaluation is _____.

Instructor shall identify by * those steps considered critical. If step is missed or minimum competency is not met, the evaluated procedure fails and must be repeated.

Performance Criteria	*	Self	Peer	Instructor	Comments
1. Identifies and attaches the low-speed hand-piece to the dental unit, ensuring that the receptors are aligned and the handpiece fits correctly onto the correct line.					
2. Identifies and attaches the contra-angle attachment onto the straight attachment of the low-speed handpiece, ensuring that the attachment is locked.					
3. Identifies and attaches the prophylaxis-angle attachment onto the straight attach-ment of the low-speed handpiece, ensuring that the attachment is locked.					
4. Identifies and attaches the high-speed handpiece to the dental unit, ensuring that the receptors are aligned and the handpiece fits correctly onto the correct line.					
5. Identifies and attaches the ultrasonic hand-piece to the dental unit, ensuring that the receptors are aligned and the handpiece fits correctly onto the correct line.					
Additional Comments					

Total number of points possible _____

Total number of points received _____

Grade _____ *Instructor's initials* _____ *Date* _____

107

Performance Objective

By following a routine procedure that meets stated protocols, when provided with the appropriate materials, the student will demonstrate the proper technique for preparing, cleaning, and sterilizing the dental handpiece.

Evaluation and Grading Criteria

3	Student competently met the stated criteria without assistance.
2	Student required assistance in order to meet the stated criteria.
1	Student showed uncertainty when performing the stated criteria.
0	Student was not prepared and needs to repeat the step.
N/A	No evaluation of this step.

Instructor shall define grades for each point range earned on completion of each performance-evaluated task.

Performance Standards

The minimum number of satisfactory performances required before final evaluation is _____.

Instructor shall identify by * those steps considered critical. If a step is missed or minimum competency is not met, the evaluated procedure fails and must be repeated.

Performance criteria	*	Self	Peer	Instructor	Comments
1. Placed personal protective equipment according to procedure.					
2. With the bur still in the chuck, wiped any visible debris from the handpiece. Operated the handpiece for approximately 10 to 20 seconds.					
3. Removed the bur from the handpiece and then removed the handpiece from the hose.					
4. Used a handpiece cleaner recommended by the manufacturer to remove internal debris and lubricated the handpiece according to the manufacturer's recommendations.					
5. Reattached the handpiece to an air hose, inserted a bur, and operated the handpiece to blow out the excess lubricant from the rotating parts.					

Performance criteria	*	Self	Peer	Instructor	Comments
6. Used a cotton-tipped applicator dampened with isopropyl alcohol to remove all excess lubricant from fiber-optic interfaces and exposed optical surfaces.					
7. Dried the handpiece and packaged it for sterilization.					

Additional Comments

Total number of points earned _____

Grade _____ Instructor's initials _____

COMPETENCY 12-7 IDENTIFYING AND ATTACHING BURS FOR ROTARY CUTTING INSTRUMENTS

Performance Objective

By following a routine procedure that meets stated protocols, the student will be able to identify and attach burs for the rotary cutting instruments.

Evaluation and Grading Criteria

3   Student competently met the stated criteria without assistance.

2   Student required assistance in order to meet the stated criteria.

1   Student showed uncertainty when performing the stated criteria.

0   Student was not prepared and needs to repeat the step.

N/A   No evaluation of this step.

Instructor shall define grades for each point range earned upon completion of each performance-evaluated task.

Performance Standards

The minimum number of satisfactory performances required prior to final evaluation is _____.

Instructor shall identify by * those steps considered critical. If step is missed or minimum competency is not met, the evaluated procedure fails and must be repeated.

Performance Criteria	*	Self	Peer	Instructor	Comments
1. Identified specific dental burs such as carbide, diamond, finishing, and abrasion burs, by their name and number sequence.					
2. Attached latch-typed burs to the contra-angle attachment on the low-speed handpiece, ensuring that the bur was locked in place.					
3. Attached friction-grip burs to the high-speed handpiece, ensuring that the bur was locked in place.					
4. Attached abrasive disks to the mandrel correctly, by screwing to tighten or by positioning the metal opening onto the mandrel, ensuring that the disk was securely locked.					

Additional Comments

Total number of points possible _____

Total number of points received _____

Grade _____ *Instructor's initials* _____ *Date* _____

13 The Dental Examination

TRUE/FALSE

_____ 1. The identification of a disease is called a *diagnosis.*

_____ 2. Dental recording or charting can be described by the dental team as "shorthand."

_____ 3. In an anatomic charting diagram, the illustration of each tooth resembles circles that are divided into segments.

_____ 4. When charting, blue, or black coding is used to represent dental treatment that needs to be completed.

_____ 5. The charting abbreviation for mesial-occlusal-distal-lingual is MODL.

_____ 6. Intraoral imaging provides a visual evaluation of bone and tissue that cannot be seen by other means.

_____ 7. Study casts are considered part of the diagnosis component of the exam.

_____ 8. The operator uses their hands in the palpation technique to examine hard and soft tissue of the mouth and face.

_____ 9. A thorough oral examination includes a careful examination of the neck, face, lips, and the soft tissues in the mouth.

_____ 10. It is common practice for the dental assistant to perform the periodontal examination for a patient.

MATCHING

_____ 11. Decay in pits and fissures on the occlusal surfaces of teeth

_____ 12. Decay, abrasion, or defects on the incisal edge of anterior teeth and occlusal surfaces of posterior teeth

_____ 13. Decay on proximal surfaces of incisors and canines

_____ 14. Smooth surface decay occurring on the gingival third of the facial or lingual surfaces

_____ 15. Decay on the proximal surfaces of premolars and molars involving two or more surfaces

_____ 16. Decay on the proximal surfaces of incisors and canines also involving the incisal angle

A. Class III

B. Class I

C. Class VI

D. Class II

E. Class IV

F. Class V

113

17. Describe the three levels of treatment plans that may be prescribed for a patient, depending on the need.

18. Name each of the charting symbols below by identifying the surface and condition (e.g., MOD amalgam).

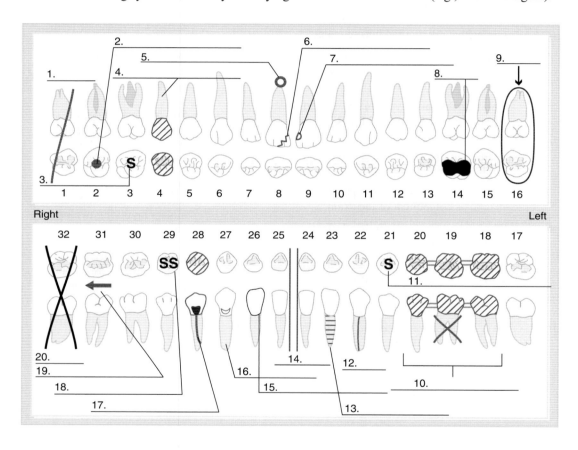

COMPETENCY 13-1 SOFT TISSUE EXAMINATION (EXPANDED FUNCTION)

Performance Objective

By following a routine procedure that meets stated protocols, the student will be able to perform a soft tissue examination.

Evaluation and Grading Criteria

3   Student competently met the stated criteria without assistance.

2   Student required assistance in order to meet the stated criteria.

1   Student showed uncertainty when performing the stated criteria.

0   Student was not prepared and needs to repeat the step.

N/A   No evaluation of this step.

Instructor shall define grades for each point range earned upon completion of each performance-evaluated task.

Performance Standards

The minimum number of satisfactory performances required prior to final evaluation is _____.

Instructor shall identify by * those steps considered critical. If step is missed or minimum competency is not met, the evaluated procedure fails and must be repeated.

Performance Criteria	*	Self	Peer	Instructor	Comments
Patient Preparation					
1. When escorting the patient to the treatment area, observes the patient's general appearance, speech, and behavior.					
2. Seats the patient in the dental chair in an upright position.					
3. Drapes the patient with a patient napkin.					
4. Explains the procedure to the patient.					
Extraoral Features					
1. Examines the face, neck, and ears for symmetry or abnormal swelling.					
2. Looks for abnormal tissue changes, skin abrasions, and discoloration.					
3. Evaluates the texture, color, and continuity of the vermilion border, the commissures of the lips, the philtrum, and the smile line.					
4. Documents all findings in the patient record.					
Cervical Lymph Nodes					
1. Positions self behind the patient and places index and middle fingers just below the patient's ears, where the temporomandibular joint (TMJ) is.					
2. Examines the right side of the neck, using the left hand to steady the patient's head. The fingers and thumb of the right hand gently follow the chain of lymph nodes downward, starting in front of the right ear and continuing to the clavicle.					

Performance Criteria	*	Self	Peer	Instructor	Comments
3. Examines the left side of the neck, using the right hand to steady the patient's head. The fingers and thumb of the left hand gently follow the chain of lymph nodes downward, starting at the front of the left ear and continuing to the clavicle.					
4. Documents all findings in the patient record.					
Temporomandibular Joint					
1. To evaluate the TMJ in centric, lateral, protrusive, and retrusive movements, gently places fingers in the external openings of the ears and asks the patient to open and close the mouth normally and then to move the jaw from side to side.					
2. To determine if there is noise in the TMJ during movement, listens as the patient opens and closes his or her mouth.					
3. Notes in the patient record any abnormalities or patient comments on pain, tenderness, or other problems related to opening and closing the mouth.					
Indications of Oral Habits					
1. Looks for indications of oral habits, such as thumb sucking, tongue-thrust swallow, mouth breathing, and tobacco use.					
2. Looks for signs of other oral habits, such as bruxism, grinding, and clenching. Indications should include abnormal wear on the teeth and problems in the TMJ.					
Interior of the Lips					
1. Asks the patient to open his or her mouth slightly.					
2. Examines the mucosa and labial frenum of the upper lip by gently retracting the lip with the thumb and index fingers.					
3. Examines the mucosa and labial frenum of the lower lip by gently retracting the lip with the thumb and index fingers.					
4. Palpates the tissue gently to detect lumps or abnormalities.					
Oral Mucosa and Tongue					
1. Palpates the tissue of the buccal mucosa gently by placing the thumb of one hand inside the mouth and the index and third fingers of the other hand on the exterior of the cheek.					
2. Examines the tissue covering the hard palate.					
3. Visually examines the buccal mucosa and the opening of Stensen's duct. A warm mouth mirror is also used to view the flow of saliva from the ducts.					

Performance Criteria	*	Self	Peer	Instructor	Comments
4. Asks the patient to extend his or her tongue and to relax it. Using sterile gauze, gently grasps the tip of the tongue and pulls it forward.					
5. Observes the dorsum (top) of the tongue for color, papillae, presence or lack of a coating, and abnormalities.					
6. Gently moves the tongue from side to side and examines the lateral (side) and ventral (underneath) surfaces.					
7. Uses a warm mouth mirror and observes the posterior area.					
8. Examines the uvula, base of the tongue, and posterior area of the mouth by placing a mouth mirror or tongue depressor firmly at the base of the tongue.					
9. With the mouth mirror firmly depressing the base of the tongue, has the patient say "ahh."					
Floor of the Mouth					
1. With the patient's mouth closed, palpates the soft tissue of the face above and below the mandible.					
2. Gently palpates the interior of the floor of the mouth by placing the index finger of one hand on the floor of the mouth and placing fingers of the other hand on the outer surface under the chin.					
3. Instructs the patient to touch the tongue to the hard palate.					
4. Notes the quantity and consistency of the flow of saliva.					
5. Documents all information accurately in the patient record.					
Additional Comments					

Total number of points possible _____

Total number of points received _____

Grade _____ *Instructor's initials* _____ *Date* _____

COMPETENCY 13-2 CHARTING OF TEETH

Performance Objective

By following a routine procedure that meets stated protocols, the student will be able to properly chart teeth.

Evaluation and Grading Criteria

3   Student competently met the stated criteria without assistance.

2   Student required assistance in order to meet the stated criteria.

1   Student showed uncertainty when performing the stated criteria.

0   Student was not prepared and needs to repeat the step.

N/A   No evaluation of this step.

Instructor shall define grades for each point range earned upon completion of each performance-evaluated task.

Performance Standards

The minimum number of satisfactory performances required prior to final evaluation is _____.

Instructor shall identify by * those steps considered critical. If step is missed or minimum competency is not met, the evaluated procedure fails and must be repeated.

Performance Criteria	*	Self	Peer	Instructor	Comments
Patient Preparation					
1. Patient is seated and draped with a patient napkin.					
2. Patient is placed in a supine position.					
Examination of the Teeth and Occlusion					
1. If using a paper chart, is equipped with black/blue and red pens/pencils, clinical examination form, and a flat surface. If using electronic chart, chart opened and keyboard covered.					
2. Transfers the mirror and explorer to the dentist. Beginning with tooth 1 and continuing to 32, the dentist examines every surface of each tooth.					
3. Throughout procedure, the air syringe is utilized to clear the mouth mirror and dry teeth.					
4. The operating light is adjusted as necessary for illumination of the area.					
5. Records the specific notations as the dentist dictates their findings.					
6. Articulating paper positioned in the holder and transfers with the paper positioned correctly for that side of the mouth to check occlusion.					

119

Performance Criteria	*	Self	Peer	Instructor	Comments
7. At the completion of the procedure, rinses and dries the patient's mouth.					
8. Documents all information accurately in the patient record, including signature and date.					
Additional Comments					

Total number of points possible _____

Total number of points received _____

Grade _____ *Instructor's initials* _____ *Date* _____

COMPETENCY 13-3 RECORDING THE COMPLETED DENTAL TREATMENT

Performance Objective

By following a routine procedure that meets stated protocols, the student will be able to record a complete dental treatment.

Evaluation and Grading Criteria

3   Student competently met the stated criteria without assistance.

2   Student required assistance in order to meet the stated criteria.

1   Student showed uncertainty when performing the stated criteria.

0   Student was not prepared and needs to repeat the step.

N/A   No evaluation of this step.

Instructor shall define grades for each point range earned upon completion of each performance-evaluated task.

Performance Standards

The minimum number of satisfactory performances required prior to final evaluation is _____.

Instructor shall identify by * those steps considered critical. If step is missed or minimum competency is not met, the evaluated procedure fails and must be repeated.

Performance Criteria	*	Self	Peer	Instructor	Comments
1. In the Date column, records the correct date including numbers in a month/date/year format.					
2. In the Progress Notes column, records all steps of the dental procedure, such as the tooth number, the surfaces of the tooth restored, the type and amount of anesthetic agent, the dental materials used, and the patient's tolerance of the appointment.					
3. If appropriate, describes the procedure that was performed with appropriate details, such as whether the tooth was prepared for a crown.					
4. After entering the completed treatment, signs the entry.					
5. Returns the completed dental record to the business office.					
Additional Comments					

Total number of points possible _____

Total number of points received _____

Grade _____ *Instructor's initials* _____ *Date* _____

14 Moisture Control

TRUE/FALSE

_____ 1. A dry angle is a triangle-shaped absorbent pad to isolate the anterior area of the mouth.

_____ 2. The anchor tooth is a term used for the tooth that holds the dental dam clamp.

_____ 3. When restoring tooth #14, cotton roll is positioned on buccal surface for moisture control.

_____ 4. A limited-area rinse is performed only at the completion of the dental procedure.

_____ 5. Depending on the procedure, the oral evacuator is held in either the thumb-to-nose grasp or the palm grasp.

_____ 6. HVE is the abbreviation for high-volume evacuator.

_____ 7. The dental dam is an isolation technique that can ensure a dry field.

_____ 8. HVE tips should be disinfected after use.

_____ 9. The saliva ejector is used to remove small amounts of saliva or water from a patient's mouth.

_____ 10. The dental dam is applied before the dentist administers the local anesthetic.

MATCHING

_____ 11. Dental dam punch

_____ 12. Dental dam stamp

_____ 13. Dental dam

_____ 14. Dental dam forceps

_____ 15. Dental dam frame

_____ 16. Dental dam clamps

_____ 17. Dental dam napkin

_____ 18. Lubricant

A. U-shaped piece of equipment to stretch the dam away from the face

B. Used to place and remove the dental dam clamp

C. Device used to create holes in the dam

D. Disposable absorbent placed between the face and dam

E. Device used to mark teeth on the dam

F. Material used to isolate teeth

G. Water-soluble substance placed on the underside of the dam

H. Piece of metal that anchors the dental dam material on the tooth.

19. List the three uses of the high-volume evacuator.

20. Describe the advantages and disadvantages of using cotton rolls for moisture control.

21. The table below shows locations of handpiece placement during a procedure for a right-handed operator. Fill in the surface of each tooth where the HVE tip is positioned.

If handpiece placement is on:	The HVE should be positioned on:
a. Facial surface of #9	_____
b. Occlusal surface of #4	_____
c. Lingual surface of #18	_____
d. Occlusal surface of #13	_____
e. Lingual surface of #24	_____
f. Buccal surface of #30	_____

22. List the indications for using the dental dam.

Performance Objective

By following a routine procedure that meets stated protocols, the student will be able to properly perform a mouth rinse on a patient.

Evaluation and Grading Criteria

3   Student competently met the stated criteria without assistance.

2   Student required assistance in order to meet the stated criteria.

1   Student showed uncertainty when performing the stated criteria.

0   Student was not prepared and needs to repeat the step.

N/A   No evaluation of this step.

Instructor shall define grades for each point range earned upon completion of each performance-evaluated task.

Performance Standards

The minimum number of satisfactory performances required prior to final evaluation is _____.

Instructor shall identify by * those steps considered critical. If step is missed or minimum competency is not met, the evaluated procedure fails and must be repeated.

Performance Criteria	*	Self	Peer	Instructor	Comments
1. Personal protective equipment placed according to procedure.					
2. Selected the oral evacuation system that is best for rinsing.					
3. Uses proper grasp of the air-water syringe in left hand, and the HVE or saliva ejector in right hand.					
Limited-Mouth Rinse 4. Turns on the suction and positions the bevel of the tip at the site for rinse.					
5. Sprays the combination of air and water onto the site to be rinsed.					
6. Suctions all fluid and debris from the area, being sure to remove all fluids.					
7. Dries the area by depressing air button only.					

125

Performance Criteria	*	Self	Peer	Instructor	Comments
Full-Mouth Rinse 8. Instructs the patient to turn toward the assistant.					
9. Turns on the HVE or saliva ejector and positions the bevel of the tip in the vestibule of the patient's left side.					
10. With the HVE or saliva ejector tip positioned, directs the air-water syringe from the patient's maxillary right going across to the left side, spraying all surfaces.					
11. Continues along the mandibular arch, following the same sequence from right to left.					
Additional Comments					

Total number of points possible _____

Total number of points received _____

Grade _____ *Instructor's initials* _____ *Date* _____

Performance Objective

By following a routine procedure that meets stated protocols, the student will be able to position the high-volume evacuator during a procedure.

Evaluation and Grading Criteria

3	Student competently met the stated criteria without assistance.
2	Student required assistance in order to meet the stated criteria.
1	Student showed uncertainty when performing the stated criteria.
0	Student was not prepared and needs to repeat the step.
N/A	No evaluation of this step.

Instructor shall define grades for each point range earned upon completion of each performance-evaluated task.

Performance Standards

The minimum number of satisfactory performances required prior to final evaluation is _____.

Instructor shall identify by ∗ those steps considered critical. If step is missed or minimum competency is not met, the evaluated procedure fails and must be repeated.

Performance Criteria	∗	Self	Peer	Instructor	Comments
1. Places the HVE tip in the holder by pushing the end of the tip into the holder through the plastic barrier.					
2. If necessary, uses the HVE tip or a mouth mirror to gently retract the cheek or tongue.					
Posterior Placement 1. For a mandibular site, places a cotton roll before placement of the suction tip.					
2. Places the bevel of the HVE tip as close as possible to the tooth being prepared.					
3. Positions the bevel of the HVE tip parallel to the buccal or lingual surface of the tooth being prepared.					
4. Places the upper edge of the HVE tip so that it extends slightly beyond the occlusal surface.					
Anterior Placement 1. If the dentist is preparing the tooth from the lingual aspect, HVE tip is positioned parallel to the facial surface and slightly beyond the incisal edge.					
2. If the dentist is preparing the tooth from the facial aspect, HVE tip is positioned parallel to the lingual surface and slightly beyond the incisal edge.					
Additional Comments					

Total number of points possible _____

Total number of points received _____

Grade _____ *Instructor's initials* _____ *Date* _____

127

COMPETENCY 14-3 PLACING AND REMOVING COTTON ROLLS

Performance Objective

By following a routine procedure that meets stated protocols, the student will be able to place and remove cotton rolls in the patient's mouth.

Evaluation and Grading Criteria

3   Student competently met the stated criteria without assistance.

2   Student required assistance in order to meet the stated criteria.

1   Student showed uncertainty when performing the stated criteria.

0   Student was not prepared and needs to repeat the step.

N/A   No evaluation of this step.

Instructor shall define grades for each point range earned upon completion of each performance-evaluated task.

Performance Standards

The minimum number of satisfactory performances required prior to final evaluation is _____.

Instructor shall identify by * those steps considered critical. If step is missed or minimum competency is not met, the evaluated procedure fails and must be repeated.

Performance Criteria	*	Self	Peer	Instructor	Comments
Maxillary Placement					
1. Instructs the patient to raise the chin and turn his or her head toward the assistant.					
2. Using the cotton pliers, picks up cotton roll so that it is positioned even with the beaks of the cotton pliers.					
3. Transfers the cotton roll to the mouth and positions it securely in the mucobuccal fold closest to the working field.					
4. This placement can be used for any location on the maxillary arch.					
Mandibular Placement					
1. Instructs the patient to turn his or her head toward the assistant with chin lowered.					
2. Using the cotton pliers, picks up cotton roll so that it is positioned even with the beaks of the pliers.					
3. Transfers the cotton roll to the mouth and positions it securely in the mucobuccal fold closest to the working field.					
4. Carries the second cotton roll to the mouth and positions it in the floor of the mouth between the working field and the tongue.					
5. For the anterior region, the cotton roll is slightly bent before placement for a better fit.					
6. If using a saliva ejector, placement is completed after cotton roll is positioned in the lingual vestibule.					

129

Performance Criteria	*	Self	Peer	Instructor	Comments
Cotton Roll Removal					
1. At the completion of procedure, removes the cotton roll before the full-mouth rinse. If the cotton roll appears dry, moistens it with water from the air-water syringe before removal.					
2. Using cotton pliers, retrieves the contaminated cotton roll from the site.					
3. If appropriate for the procedure, performs a limited rinse.					
Additional Comments					

Total number of points possible _____

Total number of points received _____

Grade _____ Instructor's initials _____ Date _____

COMPETENCY 14-4 PREPARATION, PLACEMENT, AND REMOVAL OF THE DENTAL DAM (EXPANDED FUNCTION)

Performance Objective

By following a routine procedure that meets stated protocols, the student will be able to prepare, place, and remove a dental dam.

Evaluation and Grading Criteria

3   Student competently met the stated criteria without assistance.

2   Student required assistance in order to meet the stated criteria.

1   Student showed uncertainty when performing the stated criteria.

0   Student was not prepared and needs to repeat the step.

N/A   No evaluation of this step.

Instructor shall define grades for each point range earned upon completion of each performance-evaluated task.

Performance Standards

The minimum number of satisfactory performances required prior to final evaluation is _____.

Instructor shall identify by * those steps considered critical. If step is missed or minimum competency is not met, the evaluated procedure fails and must be repeated.

Performance Criteria	*	Self	Peer	Instructor	Comments
1. Personal protective equipment placed according to procedure.					
2. Obtained set-up for dental dam.					
Patient Preparation					
1. Reviews the patient's record for any contraindications to using a dental dam.					
2. Identifies the area to be isolated. Informs the patient of the need to place a dental dam and explains the steps involved.					
3. Assists the dentist in the administration of local anesthetic. The operator determines which teeth are to be isolated and notes whether there are any malposed teeth to be accommodated.					
4. Applies lubricating ointment to the patient's lip with a cotton roll or cotton-tip applicator.					
5. Uses the mouth mirror and explorer to examine the site where the dam is to be placed. Makes sure it is free of plaque and debris.					
6. Flosses all contacts involved before placement of the dental dam.					
Punching the Dental Dam					
7. Uses a template or stamp to mark on the dam the isolated teeth.					
8. Correctly punches the dam according to the teeth to be isolated. Uses the correct size of punch hole for each specific tooth.					

131

Performance Criteria	*	Self	Peer	Instructor	Comments
9. If there are tight contacts, lightly lubricates the punched holes on the undersurface of the dam.					
Placing the Clamp and Frame 10. Selects the correct size of clamp.					
11. Secures the clamp by tying a ligature of dental tape around the bow of the clamp.					
12. Places the beaks of the rubber dam forceps into the holes of the clamp. Grasps the handles of the rubber dam forceps and squeezes to open the clamp. Turns upward and allows the locking bar to slide down to keep the forceps open for placement.					
13. Positions himself or herself in the operator's position and adjusts the patient for easier access.					
14. Retrieves the rubber dam forceps. Positions the lingual jaws of the clamp first, then the facial jaws. During placement, keeps an index finger on the clamp to prevent the clamp from coming off before it is stabilized on the tooth. Checks the clamp for fit.					
15. Transfers the dental dam to the site; stretches the punched hole for the anchor tooth over the clamp.					
16. Using cotton pliers, retrieves the ligature and pulls it through so that it is exposed and easy to grasp if necessary.					
17. Positions the frame over the dam and slightly pulls the dam, allowing it to hook onto the projections of the frame.					
18. Fits the last hole of the dam over the last tooth exposed at the opposite end of the anchor tooth.					
19. Using the index fingers of both hands, stretches the dam on the lingual and facial surfaces of the teeth so that the dam slides through each contact area.					
20. With a piece of dental tape or waxed floss, flosses through each contact, pushing the dam below the proximal contacts of each tooth to be isolated.					
21. If the contacts are extremely tight, uses floss in the interproximal area to separate the teeth slightly.					
22. A ligature is placed to stabilize the dam at the opposite end of the anchor tooth.					
Inverting the Dam 1. Inverts or reverses the dam by gently stretching it near the cervix of the tooth.					
2. Applies air from the air-water syringe to the tooth being inverted to help in turning the dam material under.					
3. Uses a black spoon or burnisher to invert the edges of the dam into the sulcus.					

132

Performance Criteria	*	Self	Peer	Instructor	Comments
4. When all punched holes are properly inverted, the dental dam application is complete.					
5. If necessary, for patient comfort, a saliva ejector is placed under the dam. This is positioned on the floor of the patient's mouth on the side opposite the area being treated.					
6. If the patient is uncomfortable and has trouble breathing through his or her nose, a piece of the dam near the palatal area is pinched with cotton pliers and a small hole is cut.					
Removing the Dam 1. If a ligature is used to stabilize the dam, removes it. If a saliva ejector is used, removes it.					
2. Slides finger under the dam parallel to the arch and pulls outward so that the holes are stretched away from the isolated teeth. Working from posterior to anterior, uses the crown and bridge scissors to cut from hole to hole, creating one long cut.					
3. When all septa are cut, pulls the dam lingually to free the rubber from the interproximal space.					
4. Using the dental dam forceps, positions the beaks into the holes of the clamp and opens the clamp by squeezing the handle. Gently slides the clamp from the tooth.					
5. Removes both the dam and the frame at one time.					
6. Uses a tissue or the dam napkin to wipe the patient's mouth and lips free of moisture.					
7. Inspects the dam to ensure that the entire pattern of the torn septa of the dental dam has been removed.					
8. If a fragment of the dental dam is missing, uses dental floss and checks the corresponding interproximal area of the oral cavity.					
Additional Comments					

Total number of points possible _____

Total number of points received _____

Grade _____ *Instructor's initials* _____ *Date* _____

15 Pain and Anxiety Management

TRUE/FALSE

_____ 1. A local anesthetic with the addition of a vasoconstrictor will cause a blood vessel to constrict.

_____ 2. An anesthetic cartridge is also referred to as a *syringe*.

_____ 3. A contraindication for receiving nitrous oxide/oxygen would be pulmonary disease in a patient.

_____ 4. In order to identify injectable local anesthetics, a color-coding system was designed using blue and green.

_____ 5. *Duration* is the time frame from when an injection is given until the numbing sensation is gone.

_____ 6. A topical anesthetic is used to provide a temporary numbing effect on the nerve endings on the surface of the oral mucosa.

_____ 7. Block anesthesia is the procedure of injecting anesthetic solution into the tissues near the apices of the tooth that is being treated.

_____ 8. The transfer of a syringe should take place in the operator's zone.

_____ 9. Analgesics are drugs that dull the perception of pain without producing unconsciousness.

_____ 10. Tylenol® is a brand name of acetaminophen.

MATCHING

Match the type of drug with its drug category.

_____ 11. Penicillin   A. Analgesic

_____ 12. Ibuprofen   B. Antibiotic

_____ 13. Morphine   C. Sedative

_____ 14. Valium   D. Narcotic

Match the following parts of the anesthetic syringe with their general description:

_____ 15. Thumb ring

_____ 16. Harpoon

_____ 17. Barrel of syringe

_____ 18. Finger grip

_____ 19. Piston rod

_____ 20. Threaded tip

A. Hub where the needle is screwed onto the syringe

B. Where the dentist holds the syringe firmly

C. Sharp, hook like-component that fits into the rubber stopper of the cartridge

D. Holds the anesthetic cartridge

E. C-shaped portion of the area grasped by the operator

F. Pushes down the rubber stopper on the anesthetic cartridge

SHORT ANSWER

21. List five specific health conditions that could affect the selection of a local anesthetic.

22. Provide three advantages of using nitrous oxide analgesia.

135

COMPETENCY 15-1 APPLYING A TOPICAL ANESTHETIC OINTMENT

Performance Objective

By following a routine procedure that meets stated protocols, the student will be able to properly apply a topical anesthetic.

Evaluation and Grading Criteria

3	Student competently met the stated criteria without assistance.
2	Student required assistance in order to meet the stated criteria.
1	Student showed uncertainty when performing the stated criteria.
0	Student was not prepared and needs to repeat the step.
N/A	No evaluation of this step.

Instructor shall define grades for each point range earned upon completion of each performance-evaluated task.

Performance Standards

The minimum number of satisfactory performances required prior to final evaluation is _____.

Instructor shall identify by * those steps considered critical. If step is missed or minimum competency is not met, the evaluated procedure fails and must be repeated.

Performance Criteria	*	Self	Peer	Instructor	Comments
1. Equipment and supplies assembled.					
Preparation 1. Readies the cotton-tipped applicator by placing a small amount of topical ointment on it. Replaces the cover of the ointment.					
2. Explains the procedure to the patient.					
3. Determines the injection site and gently dries the site with a gauze square.					
Placement 1. Places the ointment directly on the injection site.					
2. Repeats above steps if multiple injections are given.					
3. Allows the applicator to remain on the site for 3-5 minutes.					
4. Removes the applicator just before the dentist gives the injection.					
Additional Comments					

Total number of points possible _____

Total number of points received _____

Grade _____ Instructor's initials _____ Date_____

Chapter **15 Pain and Anxiety Management**

COMPETENCY 15-2 ASSEMBLING THE LOCAL ANESTHETIC SYRINGE

Performance Objective

By following a routine procedure that meets stated protocols, the student will be able to assemble a local anesthetic syringe.

Evaluation and Grading Criteria

3   Student competently met the stated criteria without assistance.

2   Student required assistance in order to meet the stated criteria.

1   Student showed uncertainty when performing the stated criteria.

0   Student was not prepared and needs to repeat the step.

N/A   No evaluation of this step.

Instructor shall define grades for each point range earned upon completion of each performance-evaluated task.

Performance Standards

The minimum number of satisfactory performances required prior to final evaluation is _____.

Instructor shall identify by * those steps considered critical. If step is missed or minimum competency is not met, the evaluated procedure fails and must be repeated.

Performance Criteria	*	Self	Peer	Instructor	Comments
1. Personal protective equipment placed according to procedure.					
Selecting the Anesthetic 1. The location of the injection will determine the needle length. The dentist determines the type of anesthetic solution.					
2. Organizes setup and positions the items at chairside out of the patient's view.					
3. Washes hands before preparing the syringe.					
Loading the Anesthetic Cartridge 1. Holds the syringe in one hand and uses the thumb ring to pull back the plunger.					
2. With the other hand, loads the anesthetic cartridge into the syringe. The stopper end is positioned first, toward the plunger.					
3. Releases the thumb ring and allows the harpoon to engage into the stopper.					
4. Uses gentle finger pressure to engage the piston forward until the harpoon is engaged into the stopper.					
5. Checks that the harpoon is securely in place and gently pulls back on the plunger.					

139

Performance Criteria	*	Self	Peer	Instructor	Comments
Placing the Needle on the Syringe					
1. Breaks the seal on the needle and removes the protective cap from the needle.					
2. Screws the needle into position on the syringe. Takes care to position the needle straight and firmly attached.					
3. Places the prepared syringe on the tray ready for use and out of the patient's sight.					
Additional Comments					

Total number of points possible _____

Total number of points received _____

Grade _____ *Instructor's initials* _____ *Date* _____

Performance Objective

By following a routine procedure that meets stated protocols, the student will be able to assist in the administration of local anesthesia.

Evaluation and Grading Criteria

3	Student competently met the stated criteria without assistance.
2	Student required assistance in order to meet the stated criteria.
1	Student showed uncertainty when performing the stated criteria.
0	Student was not prepared and needs to repeat the step.
N/A	No evaluation of this step.

Instructor shall define grades for each point range earned upon completion of each performance-evaluated task.

Performance Standards

The minimum number of satisfactory performances required prior to final evaluation is _____.

Instructor shall identify by * those steps considered critical. If step is missed or minimum competency is not met, the evaluated procedure fails and must be repeated.

Performance Criteria	*	Self	Peer	Instructor	Comments
1. Personal protective equipment placed according to procedure.					
2. Applies topical anesthetic to the appropriate area of injection.					
3. Loosens the needle guard.					
4. Transfers the syringe in the transfer zone, just below chin out of sight of patient.					
5. Places the thumb ring over the dentist's thumb, making sure syringe is secure in the operator's hand.					
6. While the dentist is giving the injection, monitors the patient for any adverse reactions and projects a calming and relaxed manner.					
7. The dentist returns the contaminated syringe to the tray and replaces the needle guard by using a one-handed scoop technique or a recapping device.					
8. After the injection, instructs the patient to turn toward the assistant. Rinses the patient's mouth with the air-water syringe, using either the high-volume evacuator or saliva ejector.					
9. Continues monitoring the patient throughout the procedure for any adverse effects.					

Performance Criteria	*	Self	Peer	Instructor	Comments
10. At the completion of the procedure, instructs the patient about the numbness and not to bite his or her lip or cheek.					
11. Before leaving the dental treatment area, removes the used needle with the needle guard still in place and disposes of it in the sharps container.					
12. Removes the anesthetic cartridge and disposes of it with the medical waste. Places the syringe on the tray to be returned to the sterilization center.					
13. Records the type and amount of anesthesia used for procedure.					

Total number of points possible _____

Total number of points received _____

Grade _____ *Instructor's initials* _____ *Date* _____

COMPETENCY 15-4 ASSISTING IN THE ADMINISTRATION AND MONITORING OF NITROUS OXIDE-OXYGEN SEDATION (EXPANDED FUNCTION)

Performance Objective

By following a routine procedure that meets stated protocols, the student will be able to assist in the administration and monitoring of nitrous oxide/oxygen sedation.

Evaluation and Grading Criteria

3   Student competently met the stated criteria without assistance.

2   Student required assistance in order to meet the stated criteria.

1   Student showed uncertainty when performing the stated criteria.

0   Student was not prepared and needs to repeat the step.

N/A   No evaluation of this step.

Instructor shall define grades for each point range earned upon completion of each performance-evaluated task.

Performance Standards

The minimum number of satisfactory performances required prior to final evaluation is _____.

Instructor shall identify by * those steps considered critical. If step is missed or minimum competency is not met, the evaluated procedure fails and must be repeated.

Performance Criteria	*	Self	Peer	Instructor	Comments
1. Checked the tanks for adequate supply of gases as part of morning preparation.					
2. Personal protective equipment placed according to procedure.					
3. Gathered appropriate supplies and placed a sterile mask of the appropriate size on the tubing.					
4. Seats the patient, updates the medical history, and takes and records vital signs.					
5. Instructs the patient on the use of nitrous oxide/oxygen with the patient.					
6. Places the patient in a supine position.					
7. Assists the patient to position the mask over his or her nose and adjusts the fit.					
8. Tightens the tubing once it is comfortable for the patient.					
9. If the mask pinches or causes discomfort, places gauze square under the edge.					

Performance Criteria	*	Self	Peer	Instructor	Comments
Administration					
1. At the dentist's instructions, begins adjusting the flow meter for O_2 flow only. The patient is given 100% oxygen for at least 1 minute.					
2. At the dentist's direction, adjusts N_2O flow in increments of 0.5 to 1 L/minute and reduces O_2 flow by a corresponding amount.					
3. At 1-minute intervals, the previous step is repeated until the dentist determines that the patient has reached the baseline reading.					
4. Records the patient's baseline level in the patient chart.					
5. Monitors the patient closely throughout the procedure.					
Oxygenation					
1. Toward the end of the procedure, N_2O is depleted and 100% O_2 is administered, as directed by the dentist.					
2. After oxygenation is complete, removes the mask. Slowly positions the patient upright.					
3. Records the patient's baseline level of N_2O and O_2 and reaction during analgesia.					
Additional Comments					

Total number of points possible _____

Total number of points received _____

Grade _____ *Instructor's initials* _____ *Date* _____

16 Principal Concepts of Radiation

TRUE/FALSE

_____ 1. When X-rays strike patient tissues, ionization occurs.

_____ 2. The amount of radiation that is absorbed by the tissues is called *dose equivalence.*

_____ 3. The maximum permissible dose (MPD) for occupationally exposed persons is 5.0 rem.

_____ 4. The fastest speed film used in dentistry is "F-Speed."

_____ 5. Collimation is used to remove the longer-wavelength, low-energy X-rays from the X-ray beam.

FILL IN THE BLANK

6. _____ is when small amounts of radiation are absorbed over a long period of time.

7. _____ is when large amounts of radiation are absorbed in a short time.

8. _____ effects of radiation are those that build up over a lifetime.

9. _____ is used to restrict the size and shape of the X-ray beam.

10. A _____ is placed over the patient's thyroid and chest during exposure to radiation.

MULTIPLE CHOICE

11. When should the dental assistant hold the film in the patient's mouth during exposure?
    a. with young children
    b. with patients with special needs
    c. with edentulous patients
    d. never

12. Images appearing dark or black on the radiograph are termed:
    a. radiolucent
    b. low contrast
    c. radiopaque
    d. distorted

13. Elongation of the image can affect:
    a. contrast
    b. density
    c. image detail
    d. all of the above

14. The milliamperage selector controls:
    a. the number of electrons that are produced
    b. the penetrating power
    c. the quality of the X-ray film
    d. all of the above

15. The exposure time for digital images is measured in units of:
    a. fractions of a second called impulses
    b. seconds
    c. minutes
    d. all of the above

LABELING

Label the parts of a dental X-ray tube.

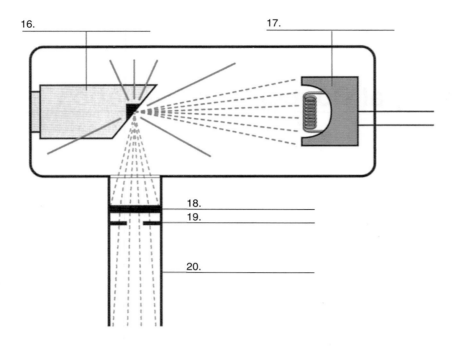

16. _____

17. _____

18. _____

19. _____

20. _____

INTERACTIVE DENTAL OFFICE PATIENT CASE EXERCISE

Access the *Interactive Dental Office* on *Evolve* and click on the patient case file for Margaret Brown.
Review Margaret's record.
Answer the following question:

1. Would it be better if the dental assistant held the film in the proper position for the child? It was only for one film.

17 Oral Radiography

TRUE/FALSE

_____ 1. The bisecting angle technique is preferred because it is more accurate than the parallel technique.

_____ 2. When using the paralleling technique, the jaw is positioned parallel to the floor while the film packet is in place.

_____ 3. In both digital and film-based techniques, the periapical radiograph is the most accurate for diagnosing dental decay.

_____ 4. In both digital and film-based techniques, incorrect horizontal angulation is responsible for closed contacts on the radiograph.

_____ 5. In both digital and film-based techniques, too little vertical angulation will cause the image to be foreshortened.

SHORT ANSWER

Describe the following stages of the automatic film processor implements to the exposed dental film.

6. Developing solution -

7. Fixing solution -

8. Water wash -

9. Drying -

Refer to **Figure 17-25** in your textbook and provide the appearance for the processing errors.

10. _____ films are caused by overdevelopment.

11. _____ films are caused by underdevelopment.

12. _____ films are caused by developer cut off.

13. _____ on the film is caused by fixer spots.

14. _____ on the film can be caused by roller marks.

15. _____ reticulation on the film.

MULTIPLE CHOICE

16. After the film has been exposed, the invisible image on the film is called the:
    a. lead foil
    b. latent image
    c. radiolucent image
    d. radiopaque image

17. How many sizes of dental film are commonly used?
    a. two
    b. three
    c. four
    d. five

18. In both digital and film-based techniques, which of the following are common sources of disease transmission during radiography procedures?
    a. X-ray machine arm, head, and position indicator device
    b. control panel and exposure button
    c. lead apron
    d. all of the above

19. Dental film should be stored in a way to protect it from:
    a. light and heat
    b. scatter radiation
    c. chemicals
    d. all of the above

20. In both digital and film-based techniques, which of the following infection control measures are not used in dental radiography?
    a. personal protective equipment (PPE)
    b. sterilization of film packets
    c. surface barriers
    d. standard operating procedures

LABELING

Identify the types of dental radiographs.

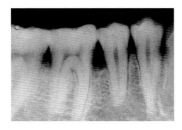

21. _____

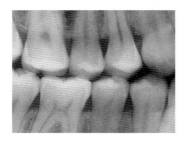

22. _____

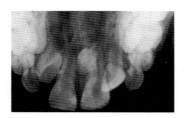

23. _____

INTERACTIVE DENTAL OFFICE PATIENT CASE EXERCISES

Access the *Interactive Dental Office* on *Evolve* and click on the patient case file for Miguel Ricardo.

Review Mr. Ricardo's record.

Mount his radiographs.

Answer the following questions:

1. Is the dark area below the roots of the mandibular molars a processing error?

2. What size film was used for the bitewings?

Access the *Interactive Dental Office* on *Evolve* and click on the patient case file for Mrs. Harriet Ross.
Review Mrs. Ross' record.
Mount her radiographs.

148

Answer the following questions:

1. Why were only 13 films taken?

2. Are there any processing errors on her FMX?

Access the *Interactive Dental Office* on *Evolve* and click on the patient case file for Mr. Lee Wong.
Review Mr. Wong's record.
Mount his radiographs.
Answer the following questions:

1. Is the dark area around the roots caused by a processing error?

2. Did a processing error cause the round circle at the bottom on the right side of the film?

Access the *Interactive Dental Office* on *Evolve* and click on the patient case file for Cindy Valladares.
Review the patient's panoramic radiograph.
Answer the following questions:

1. Were the dark areas over the roots of the mandibular teeth most likely caused by a processing error or by a positioning error?

2. Is this radiograph diagnostically acceptable? Why or why not?

Access the *Interactive Dental Office* on *Evolve* and click on the patient case file for Tiffany Cole.
Review the patient's panoramic radiograph.
Answer the following questions:

1. Based on the development of Tiffany's teeth, how old do you think she is?

2. The panoramic radiograph indicates that tooth #27 is impacted. Click on tooth #27.

Access the *Interactive Dental Office* on *Evolve* and click on the patient case file for Christopher Brooks.
Review Christopher's file.
Mount his radiographs.
Answer the following questions:

1. What types of projections were used for his radiographic survey?

2. What sizes of film were used for each projection?

Access the *Interactive Dental Office* on *Evolve* and click on the patient case file for Antonio DeAngelis.

Review Mr. DeAngelis's file.
Mount his radiographs.
Answer the following questions:

1. What technique error occurred on the mandibular left premolar exposure?

2. What is wrong with the maxillary left molar projection?

3. What is wrong with the right premolar bitewing, and what would be the correction?

With the first patient, allow yourself 5 minutes. Time yourself and note how many errors you make when you are placing these on the mount. Continue this practice until you have your mounting skills down to 2 minutes with no errors.

COMPETENCY 17-1 PRACTICING INFECTION CONTROL WITH DIGITAL SENSORS

Performance Objective

By following a routine procedure that meets stated protocols, the student will be able to perform all infection control practices using digital sensor exposure.

Evaluation and Grading Criteria

3   Student competently met the stated criteria without assistance.

2   Student required assistance in order to meet the stated criteria.

1   Student showed uncertainty when performing the stated criteria.

0   Student was not prepared and needs to repeat the step.

N/A   No evaluation of this step.

Instructor shall define grades for each point range earned upon completion of each performance-evaluated task.

Performance Standards

The minimum number of satisfactory performances required prior to final evaluation is _____.

Instructor shall identify by * those steps considered critical. If step is missed or minimum competency is not met, the evaluated procedure fails and must be repeated.

Performance Criteria	*	Self	Peer	Instructor	Comments
1. Washes and dries hands.					
2. Places surface barriers on equipment, computer keyboard and mouse, and work area.					
3. Sets out the packaged positioning device barriers for the sensor and cable, a paper towel or gauze squares, and miscellaneous items.					
4. Secures the barrier around the digital sensor.					
5. Seats the patient and places the lead apron.					
6. Washes and dries hands and applies gloves.					
7. After all the exposures are complete, removes the lead apron and dismisses the patient.					
8. Puts on utility gloves and removes barriers from the X-ray equipment, taking care not to touch the surfaces underneath.					
9. Disposes of barriers and paper towels.					
10. Places the positioning device on a tray to be returned to the instrument processing area.					
11. Disinfects the lead apron and any surfaces that may be contaminated during the removal of surface barriers.					

151

Performance Criteria	*	Self	Peer	Instructor	Comments
12. Carefully disinfects the sensor according to the manufacturer's recommendations.					
13. Washes and dries hands.					
Additional Comments					

Total number of points possible _____

Total number of points received _____

Grade _____ *Instructor's initials* _____ *Date* _____

COMPETENCY 17-2 PRACTICING INFECTION CONTROL WITH PHOSPHOR STORAGE PLATES

Performance Objective

By following a routine procedure that meets stated protocols, the student will be able to perform all infection control practices when using phosphor storage plates.

Evaluation and Grading Criteria

3   Student competently met the stated criteria without assistance.

2   Student required assistance in order to meet the stated criteria.

1   Student showed uncertainty when performing the stated criteria.

0   Student was not prepared and needs to repeat the step.

N/A   No evaluation of this step.

Instructor shall define grades for each point range earned upon completion of each performance-evaluated task.

Performance Standards

The minimum number of satisfactory performances required prior to final evaluation is _____.

Instructor shall identify by * those steps considered critical. If step is missed or minimum competency is not met, the evaluated procedure fails and must be repeated.

Performance Criteria	*	Self	Peer	Instructor	Comments
1. Turned on the computer.					
2. Logged on to link the patient's images to his or her chart.					
3. Chose the image layout to use.					
4. Washed and dried hands.					
5. Placed surface barriers on equipment and work area.					
6. Slid the phosphor plates into barrier envelopes. Sealed barrier by removing the protective strip and gently pressed to seal the edge.					
7. Set out the packaged positioning device, paper cup, transfer box, paper towel, and other miscellaneous items you might have needed.					
Exposures					
1. Seated the patient and placed the lead apron.					
2. Washed and dried hands and donned gloves.					
3. Placed the PSP into the film holder for each exposure.					
4. After each exposure, wiped excess saliva from the PSP envelope using a paper towel.					
5. Placed each exposed PSP into the paper cup labeled with the patient's name or directly into the black transfer box.					

Performance Criteria	*	Self	Peer	Instructor	Comments
6. After the exposures were complete, removed the lead apron and dismissed the patient.					
7. While still gloved, removed barriers taking care not to touch the surfaces underneath.					
8. Disposed of barriers and paper towels.					
9. Placed the used positioning device on a tray to be returned to the instrument processing area.					
Preparing PSPs for Scanning					
1. While gloved, removed each PSP from the paper cup and carefully opened the sealed envelope and allowed the PSP to drop into the black transfer box. Used care not to touch the outside of the transfer box to avoid contamination.					
2. Disposed of contaminated envelopes.					
3. Removed gloves and washed and dried hands.					
Scanning the PSP					
1. Read the specific instructions for the specific machine used.					
2. Inserted the PSP into the scanner according to the manufacturer's instructions.					
3. When the imaging was complete, logged off the system.					
4. Documented the procedure in the patient's record.					
Additional Comments					

Total number of points possible _____

Total number of points received _____

Grade _____ *Instructor's initials* _____ *Date* _____

COMPETENCY 17-3 PRACTICING INFECTION CONTROL DURING FILM EXPOSURE

NOTE: Regardless of whether you are using film, phosphor storage plates (PSPs), or digital sensors, proper infection control measures are critical.

Performance Objective

By following a routine procedure that meets stated protocols, the student will be able to perform all infection control practices during film exposure.

Evaluation and Grading Criteria

3   Student competently met the stated criteria without assistance.

2   Student required assistance in order to meet the stated criteria.

1   Student showed uncertainty when performing the stated criteria.

0   Student was not prepared and needs to repeat the step.

N/A   No evaluation of this step.

Instructor shall define grades for each point range earned upon completion of each performance-evaluated task.

Performance Standards

The minimum number of satisfactory performances required prior to final evaluation is _____.

Instructor shall identify by * those steps considered critical. If step is missed or minimum competency is not met, the evaluated procedure fails and must be repeated.

Performance Criteria	*	Self	Peer	Instructor	Comments
1. Washes and dries hands.					
2. Places surface barriers on equipment and work area.					
3. Sets out the packaged film/sensor-holding device, film, labeled container for exposed film, paper towel, and other miscellaneous items needed.					
4. Seats the patient and places the lead apron.					
5. Washes and dries hands and applies gloves.					
6. After each exposure, wipes the excess saliva from the film/sensor using a paper towel.					
7. Places each exposed film or phosphor storage plate (PSP) into the container, being careful not to touch the external surface.					
8. After exposures are complete, removes the lead apron and dismisses the patient.					
9. While still gloved, removes barriers, taking care not to touch the surfaces underneath.					
10. Disposes of barriers and paper towels.					

Performance Criteria	*	Self	Peer	Instructor	Comments
11. Places the film/sensor-holding device on a tray to be returned to the instrument processing area.					
12. Washes and dries hands.					
13. Takes the exposed films to the processing area.					
Additional Comments					

Total number of points possible _____

Total number of points received _____

Grade _____ *Instructor's initials* _____ *Date* _____

COMPETENCY 17-4 ASSEMBLING EXTENSION-CONE PARALLELING (XCP) INSTRUMENTS

NOTE: There are specific XCP instruments for digital sensors and for film. Both types designate blue for anterior placement and yellow for posterior placement.

Performance Objective

By following a routine procedure that meets stated protocols, the student will be able to assemble the Rinn XCP instruments for all areas of the mouth in preparation for radiographic surveys.

Evaluation and Grading Criteria

3   Student competently met the stated criteria without assistance.

2   Student required assistance in order to meet the stated criteria.

1   Student showed uncertainty when performing the stated criteria.

0   Student was not prepared and needs to repeat the step.

N/A   No evaluation of this step.

Instructor shall define grades for each point range earned upon completion of each performance-evaluated task.

Performance Standards

The minimum number of satisfactory performances required prior to final evaluation is _____.

Instructor shall identify by * those steps considered critical. If step is missed or minimum competency is not met, the evaluated procedure fails and must be repeated.

Performance Criteria	*	Self	Peer	Instructor	Comments
Anterior Assembly					
1. Lays out the blue parts for the anterior XCP instrument.					
2. Assembles the anterior XCP instrument by inserting the two prongs of the blue anterior indicator arm into the openings in the blue anterior bite-block.					
3. Inserts the blue anterior indicator arm into the opening on the blue anterior aiming ring.					
4. Flexes the plastic backing of the blue bite-block to open the film slot for easy insertion of the anterior film packet.					
5. The blue anterior XCP instrument is correctly assembled when the film is seen centered in the middle of the aiming ring.					
Posterior Assembly					
1. Lays out the yellow parts for the posterior XCP instrument.					
2. Assembles the posterior XCP instrument by inserting the two prongs of the yellow posterior indicator arm into the openings in the yellow posterior bite-block.					

Performance Criteria	*	Self	Peer	Instructor	Comments
3. Inserts the yellow posterior indicator arm into the opening on the yellow posterior aiming ring.					
4. Flexes the plastic backing of the yellow bite-block to open the film slot for easy insertion of the posterior film packet.					
5. The yellow posterior XCP instrument is correctly assembled when the film is centered in the middle of the aiming ring.					
Additional Comments					

Total number of points possible _____

Total number of points received _____

Grade _____ *Instructor's initials* _____ *Date* _____

COMPETENCY 17-5 PRODUCING A FULL-MOUTH RADIOGRAPHIC SURVEY USING THE PARALLELING TECHNIQUE

Performance Objective

By following a routine procedure that meets stated protocols, the student will be able to follow the proper steps to produce an FMX using the paralleling technique.

Evaluation and Grading Criteria

3   Student competently met the stated criteria without assistance.

2   Student required assistance in order to meet the stated criteria.

1   Student showed uncertainty when performing the stated criteria.

0   Student was not prepared and needs to repeat the step.

N/A   No evaluation of this step.

Instructor shall define grades for each point range earned upon completion of each performance-evaluated task.

Performance Standards

The minimum number of satisfactory performances required prior to final evaluation is _____.

Instructor shall identify by * those steps considered critical. If step is missed or minimum competency is not met, the evaluated procedure fails and must be repeated.

Performance Criteria	*	Self	Peer	Instructor	Comments
Preparation Before Seating Patient					
1. Prepares the operatory with infection control barriers.					
2. Determines the number and type of views to be exposed by reviewing the patient's chart, as pre-scribed by the dentist.					
3. If using either film or PSPs, labels a paper cup with the patient's name and date.					
4. Turns on the X-ray machine and checks the basic set-tings (kilovoltage, milliamperage, and exposure time).					
5. Washes and dries hands.					
6. Dispenses the desired number of films, and stores them outside the room where the X-ray machine is being used.					
Positioning Patient					
1. Seats the patient comfortably in the dental chair, with the back in an upright position and head supported.					
2. Asks the patient to remove eyeglasses and bulky earrings.					
3. Asks the patient to remove prosthetic appliances or objects from the mouth.					
4. Positions the patient with the occlusal plane of the jaw being imaged parallel to the floor when the mouth is open.					
5. Drapes the patient with a lead apron and thyroid collar.					

159

Performance Criteria	*	Self	Peer	Instructor	Comments
6. Washes and dries hands, then dons clean examination gloves.					
7. Opens the package and assembles the sterile film/sensor-holding instruments.					
Maxillary Canine Region					
1. Inserts the No. 1 film packet or sensor vertically into the anterior bite-block.					
2. Positions the film packet or sensor with the canine and first premolar centered. Positions the film/sensor as far posterior in the mouth as possible.					
3. With the film/sensor-holding instrument and film in place, instructs the patient to close his or her mouth slowly and firmly.					
4. Positions the localizing ring and position indicating device (PID); takes exposure.					
Maxillary Central/Lateral Incisor Region					
1. Inserts the No. 1 film packet or sensor vertically into the anterior block.					
2. Centers the film packet or sensor between the central and lateral incisors. Positions the film/sensor as far posterior in the mouth as possible.					
3. With the instrument and film in place, instructs the patient to close his or her mouth slowly and firmly.					
4. Positions the localizing ring and PID; takes exposure.					
Mandibular Canine Region					
1. Inserts the No. 1 film packet or sensor vertically into the anterior block.					
2. Centers the film/sensor on the canine. Positions the film/sensor as far in the lingual direction as the patient's anatomy allows.					
3. With the instrument and film in place, instructs the patient to close his or her mouth slowly and firmly.					
4. Positions the localizing ring and PID; takes exposure.					
Mandibular Incisor Region					
1. Inserts the No. 1 film packet or sensor vertically into the anterior bite-block.					
2. Centers the film/sensor packet between the central incisors. Positions the film/sensor as far in the lingual direction as the patient's anatomy allows.					
3. With the instrument and film in place, instructs the patient to close his or her mouth slowly and firmly.					

Performance Criteria	*	Self	Peer	Instructor	Comments
4. Slides the localizing ring to the patient's skin surface.					
5. Positions the localizing ring and the PID; takes exposure.					
Maxillary Premolar Region					
1. Inserts the film/sensor horizontally into the posterior bite-block, pushing the film/sensor to the slot.					
2. Centers the film/sensor on the second premolar. Positions the film in the mid-palate area.					
3. With the instrument and film in place, instructs the patient to close his or her mouth slowly and firmly.					
4. Positions the localizing ring and PID; takes exposure.					
Maxillary Molar Region					
1. Inserts the film/sensor horizontally into the posterior bite-block.					
2. Centers the film/sensor on the second molar. Positions the film/sensor in the mid-palate area.					
3. With the instrument and film in place, instructs the patient to close his or her mouth slowly and firmly.					
4. Positions the localizing ring and PID; takes exposure.					
Mandibular Premolar Region					
1. Inserts the No. 2 film/sensor horizontally into the posterior bite-block.					
2. Centers the film/sensor on the contact point between the second premolar and first molar. Positions the film/sensor as far lingual as the patient's anatomy allows.					
3. With instrument and film in place, instructs the patient to close his or her mouth slowly and firmly.					
4. Slides the localizing ring to the patient's skin surface.					
5. Positions the localizing ring and the PID; takes exposure.					
Mandibular Molar Region					
1. Inserts the No. 2 film/sensor horizontally into the posterior bite-block.					
2. Centers the film/sensor on the second molar. Positions the film/sensor as far lingual as the patient's anatomy allows.					
3. With the instrument and film in place, instructs the patient to close his or her mouth slowly and firmly.					

161

Performance Criteria	*	Self	Peer	Instructor	Comments
4. Slides the localizing ring to the patient's skin surface.					
5. Positions the localizing ring and PID; takes exposure.					
Additional Comments					

Total number of points possible _____

Total number of points received _____

Grade _____ Instructor's initials _____ Date _____

COMPETENCY 17-6 PRODUCING A FOUR-FILM RADIOGRAPHIC SURVEY USING THE BITE-WING TECHNIQUE

Performance Objective

By following a routine procedure that meets stated protocols, the student will be able to produce a four-view series of radiographs using the bite-wing technique.

Evaluation and Grading Criteria

3	Student competently met the stated criteria without assistance.
2	Student required assistance in order to meet the stated criteria.
1	Student showed uncertainty when performing the stated criteria.
0	Student was not prepared and needs to repeat the step.
N/A	No evaluation of this step.

Instructor shall define grades for each point range earned upon completion of each performance-evaluated task.

Performance Standards

The minimum number of satisfactory performances required prior to final evaluation is _____.

Instructor shall identify by ∗ those steps considered critical. If step is missed or minimum competency is not met, the evaluated procedure fails and must be repeated.

Performance Criteria	∗	Self	Peer	Instructor	Comments
Premolar Bite-Wing Exposure					
1. Sets vertical angulation at 10 degrees.					
2. Positions the patient with the occlusal plane parallel to the floor by instructing the patient to lower or raise his or her chin.					
3. Positions the film/sensor in the patient's mouth by placing the lower half between the tongue and mandibular teeth. Positions the film/sensor with the anterior border at the middle of the canine.					
4. Holds the film/sensor in place by pressing the tab over the occlusal aspect of the mandibular teeth.					
5. Asks the patient to close his or her mouth slowly, taking care not to close on the fingertip of glove.					
6. Does not pull the film/sensor too tightly against the lower teeth as the patient closes mouth.					
7. Stands in front of patient to set the horizontal angulations. To better visualize the curvature of the arch, places index finger along the premolar area. Aligns the open end of the PID parallel with index finger and the curvature of the arch in the premolar area.					
Molar Bite-Wing Exposure					
1. Sets vertical angulation at 10 degrees.					
2. Positions the patient with occlusal plane parallel to the floor by instructing the patient to lower or raise his or her chin.					

163

Performance Criteria	*	Self	Peer	Instructor	Comments
3. Positions the film in the patient's mouth by placing the lower half between the tongue and mandibular teeth. Centers the film/sensor on the second molar; the front edge of the film/sensor is aligned with the middle of the mandibular second premolar.					
4. Holds the film/sensor in place by pressing the tab over the occlusal aspect of the mandibular teeth.					
5. Asks the patient to close his or her mouth slowly, taking care not to close on the fingertip of glove.					
6. Does not pull the film too tightly against the lower teeth as the patient closes mouth.					
7. Stands in front of the patient to set the horizontal angulation. To better visualize the curvature of the arch, places index finger along the premolar area. Aligns the open end of the PID parallel with index finger and the curvature of the arch in the molar area.					
8. Makes certain that the PID is positioned far enough forward to cover both the maxillary and the mandibular canines to prevent a cone cut.					
9. Directs the central ray (CR) through the contact areas.					
10. Takes the exposure.					

Additional Comments

Total number of points possible _____

Total number of points received _____

Grade _____ *Instructor's initials* _____ *Date* _____

COMPETENCY 17-7 PRODUCING MAXILLARY AND MANDIBULAR RADIOGRAPHS USING THE OCCLUSAL TECHNIQUE

Performance Objective

By following a routine procedure that meets stated protocols, the student will be able to follow the steps of the occlusal technique in producing diagnostic-quality maxillary and mandibular x-ray films.

Evaluation and Grading Criteria

3   Student competently met the stated criteria without assistance.

2   Student required assistance in order to meet the stated criteria.

1   Student showed uncertainty when performing the stated criteria.

0   Student was not prepared and needs to repeat the step.

N/A   No evaluation of this step.

Instructor shall define grades for each point range earned upon completion of each performance-evaluated task.

Performance Standards

The minimum number of satisfactory performances required prior to final evaluation is _____.

Instructor shall identify by * those steps considered critical. If step is missed or minimum competency is not met, the evaluated procedure fails and must be repeated.

Performance Criteria	*	Self	Peer	Instructor	Comments
Maxillary Occlusal Technique					
1. Asks the patient to remove any prosthetic appliances or objects from the mouth.					
2. Places the lead apron and thyroid collar.					
3. Positions the patient's head so the film plane is parallel to the floor and mid-sagittal plane perpendicular to the floor.					
4. Places the film packet in the patient's mouth with the white side of the film on the occlusal surfaces of the maxillary teeth. The long edge of the film is placed in a side-to-side direction.					
5. Places the film as far posterior as possible.					
6. Positions the PID so the CR is directed at 65 degrees through the center of the film. The top edge of the PID is placed between the eyebrows on the bridge of the nose.					
7. Presses the X-ray machine activating button and takes exposure.					
8. Documents the procedure.					
Mandibular Occlusal Technique					
1. Reclines the patient and positions his or her head with the mid-sagittal plane perpendicular to the floor.					

Performance Criteria	*	Self	Peer	Instructor	Comments
2. Places the film packet in the patient's mouth with the white side of the film on the occlusal surfaces of the mandibular teeth. The long edge of the film is placed in a side-to-side direction.					
3. Positions the film as far posterior on the mandible as possible.					
4. Positions the PID so that the CR is directed at a 90-degree angle to the center of the film packet. The PID should have been centered about 1 inch below the chin.					
5. Presses the X-ray machine activating button and takes exposure.					
6. Documents the procedure.					
Additional Comments					

Total number of points possible _____

Total number of points received _____

Grade _____ Instructor's initials _____ Date _____

COMPETENCY 17-8 PRACTICING INFECTION CONTROL IN THE DARKROOM

Performance Objective

By following a routine procedure that meets stated protocols, the student will be able to practice infection control measures when in the darkroom.

Evaluation and Grading Criteria

3   Student competently met the stated criteria without assistance.

2   Student required assistance in order to meet the stated criteria.

1   Student showed uncertainty when performing the stated criteria.

0   Student was not prepared and needs to repeat the step.

N/A   No evaluation of this step.

Instructor shall define grades for each point range earned upon completion of each performance-evaluated task.

Performance Standards

The minimum number of satisfactory performances required prior to final evaluation is _____.

Instructor shall identify by * those steps considered critical. If step is missed or minimum competency is not met, the evaluated procedure fails and must be repeated.

Performance Criteria	*	Self	Peer	Instructor	Comments
1. Places a paper towel and a clean cup on the counter near the processor.					
2. Washes hands and dons a new pair of gloves, preferably the type that does not contain powder.					
3. Turns on the safety light, then turns off the white light. Opens the film packets and allows each exposed film to drop onto the paper towel. Is careful the unwrapped film does not come into contact with the gloves.					
4. Removes the lead foil from the packet and places into the foil-recycling container.					
5. Places the empty film packets into the clean cup.					
6. Discards the cup. Removes gloves by turning them inside out, then discards them.					
7. Places the films into the processor or on developing racks with bare hands.					
Additional Comments					

Total number of points possible _____

Total number of points received _____

Grade _____ Instructor's initials _____ Date _____

Performance Objective

By following a routine procedure that meets stated protocols, the student will be able to practice infection control measures when using the daylight loader in processing dental radiograph films.

Evaluation and Grading Criteria

3   Student competently met the stated criteria without assistance.

2   Student required assistance in order to meet the stated criteria.

1   Student showed uncertainty when performing the stated criteria.

0   Student was not prepared and needs to repeat the step.

N/A   No evaluation of this step.

Instructor shall define grades for each point range earned upon completion of each performance-evaluated task.

Performance Standards

The minimum number of satisfactory performances required prior to final evaluation is _____.

Instructor shall identify by * those steps considered critical. If step is missed or minimum competency is not met, the evaluated procedure fails and must be repeated.

Performance Criteria	*	Self	Peer	Instructor	Comments
1. Washes and dries hands; places a paper towel or piece of plastic as a barrier to cover the bottom of the daylight loader.					
2. Places the following into the bottom of the daylight loader: the cup containing the contaminated film, a clean pair of gloves, and a second empty paper cup. Then closes the top.					
3. Inserts clean hands through the sleeves of the daylight loader, then puts on gloves.					
4. Opens the packets and allows the films to drop onto the clean barrier.					
5. Places the contaminated packets into the second cup and places the lead foil into the foil container.					
6. After opening the last packet, removes gloves by turning them inside out. Inserts the films into the developing slots.					
7. After inserting the last film, pulls ungloved hands through the sleeves.					
8. Opens the top of the loader, then carefully pulls the ends of the barrier over the paper cup, used gloves, and discards.					

Additional Comments

Total number of points possible _____

Total number of points received _____

Grade _____ *Instructor's initials* _____ *Date* _____

Performance Objective

By following a routine procedure that meets stated protocols, the student will be able to process dental radiograph films using a manual tank.

Evaluation and Grading Criteria

3	Student competently met the stated criteria without assistance.
2	Student required assistance in order to meet the stated criteria.
1	Student showed uncertainty when performing the stated criteria.
0	Student was not prepared and needs to repeat the step.
N/A	No evaluation of this step.

Instructor shall define grades for each point range earned upon completion of each performance-evaluated task.

Performance Standards

The minimum number of satisfactory performances required prior to final evaluation is _____.

Instructor shall identify by * those steps considered critical. If step is missed or minimum competency is not met, the evaluated procedure fails and must be repeated.

Performance Criteria	*	Self	Peer	Instructor	Comments
Preparation					
1. Follows infection control steps.					
2. Stirs the solutions with the corresponding paddle.					
3. Checks the temperature of the solutions and refers to the processing chart to determine the times.					
4. Labels the film rack with the patient's name and date of exposure.					
5. Turns on the safelight, then turns off the white light.					
6. Washes hands and puts on gloves.					
7. Opens the film packets and allows the films to drop onto the clean paper towel. Takes care not to touch the films.					
Processing					
1. Attaches each film to the film rack with films parallel and not touching each other.					
2. Immerses the film rack in the developer solution, agitating the rack slightly.					
3. Sets and starts timer according to the recommendations stated on the processing chart.					
4. When the timer goes off, removes the rack of films and rinses in the circulating water in the center rank for 20-30 seconds. Lets the excess water drip off the films.					
5. Inserts the rack of films into the fixer tank and sets timer for 10 minutes.					

171

Performance Criteria	*	Self	Peer	Instructor	Comments
6. Returns rack of films to the center tank of circulating water for at least 20 minutes.					
7. Removes rack of films from the water and places in the film dryer. If a film dryer is not available, hangs films to air dry.					
8. When the films are completely dry, removes them from the rack and mounts and labels them.					
Additional Comments					

Total number of points possible _____

Total number of points received _____

Grade _____ Instructor's initials _____ Date _____

COMPETENCY 17-11 AUTOMATIC PROCESSING OF DENTAL RADIOGRAPHS USING THE DAYLIGHT LOADER

Performance Objective

By following a routine procedure that meets stated protocols, the student will be able to automatically process dental radiographs using a daylight loader.

Evaluation and Grading Criteria

3   Student competently met the stated criteria without assistance.

2   Student required assistance in order to meet the stated criteria.

1   Student showed uncertainty when performing the stated criteria.

0   Student was not prepared and needs to repeat the step.

N/A   No evaluation of this step.

Instructor shall define grades for each point range earned upon completion of each performance-evaluated task.

Performance Standards

The minimum number of satisfactory performances required prior to final evaluation is _____.

Instructor shall identify by * those steps considered critical. If step is missed or minimum competency is not met, the evaluated procedure fails and must be repeated.

Performance Criteria	*	Self	Peer	Instructor	Comments
1. At the beginning of the work day, turns on the machine and allows the chemicals to warm up according to the manufacturer's recommendations.					
2. Follows the infection control steps.					
3. Washes and dries hands.					
4. Opens the lid on the daylight loader and places a paper towel over the bottom. Then places two disposable cups on the towel.					
5. Puts on clean gloves and slides gloved hands through the sleeves of the daylight loader.					
6. Removes the film from its packet and checks that the black paper has not stuck to the film.					
7. Feeds the film into the machine.					
8. While the film is feeding into the machine, removes the lead foil from the packet and places it in one of the disposable cups. Drops the empty packet onto the paper towel.					
9. Keeps the films straight as they are fed slowly into the machine. Allows at least 10 seconds between insertion of each film into the processor and the insertion of the next film. Places films in the alternate film slots when possible.					

Performance Criteria	*	Self	Peer	Instructor	Comments
10. With the last film inserted into the machine, carefully removes gloves and drops them into the center of the paper towel, touching only the corners and underside of the paper towel. Wraps the paper towel over the contaminated film packets and gloves. Places the wrapped paper towel into the second cup.					
11. Removes the cup containing the lead foil and disposes of it in the recycling container.					
12. Removes the processed radiographs from the film recovery slot on the outside of the automatic processor. Allows 4-6 minutes for the automated process to be completed.					
Additional Comments					

Total number of points possible _____

Total number of points received _____

Grade _____ *Instructor's initials* _____ *Date* _____

COMPETENCY 17-12 MOUNTING DENTAL RADIOGRAPHS

Performance Objective

By following a routine procedure that meets stated protocols, the student will be able to mount a full-mouth series of dental radiographs.

Evaluation and Grading Criteria

3	Student competently met the stated criteria without assistance.
2	Student required assistance in order to meet the stated criteria.
1	Student showed uncertainty when performing the stated criteria.
0	Student was not prepared and needs to repeat the step.
N/A	No evaluation of this step.

Instructor shall define grades for each point range earned upon completion of each performance-evaluated task.

Performance Standards

The minimum number of satisfactory performances required prior to final evaluation is _____.

Instructor shall identify by * those steps considered critical. If step is missed or minimum competency is not met, the evaluated procedure fails and must be repeated.

Performance Criteria	*	Self	Peer	Instructor	Comments
1. Places a clean paper towel over the work surface in front of the viewbox.					
2. Turns on the viewbox.					
3. Labels and dates the film mount.					
4. Washes and dries hands.					
5. Identifies the embossed dot on each radiograph; places the film on the work surface with the dot facing up.					
6. Sorts the radiographs into three groups: bite-wing, anterior periapical, and posterior periapical views.					
7. Arranges the radiographs on the work surface in anatomical order. Uses knowledge of normal anatomical landmarks to distinguish maxillary from mandibular radiographs.					
8. Arranges all maxillary radiographs with the roots pointing upward and all mandibular radiographs with the roots pointing downward.					
9. Places each film in the corresponding window of the film mount. The following order for film mounting is suggested: a. Maxillary anterior periapical films b. Mandibular anterior periapical films c. Bite-wing films d. Maxillary posterior periapical films e. Mandibular posterior periapical films					

175

Performance Criteria	*	Self	Peer	Instructor	Comments
10. Checks the mounted radiographs to ensure that (a) the dots are all oriented properly, (b) the films are arranged properly in anatomical order, and (c) the films are secure in the mount.					
Additional Comments					

Total number of points possible _____

Total number of points received _____

Grade _____ *Instructor's initials* _____ *Date* _____

Performance Objective

By following a routine procedure that meets stated protocols, the student will be able to prepare the equipment necessary for a panoramic radiograph.

Evaluation and Grading Criteria

3   Student competently met the stated criteria without assistance.

2   Student required assistance in order to meet the stated criteria.

1   Student showed uncertainty when performing the stated criteria.

0   Student was not prepared and needs to repeat the step.

N/A   No evaluation of this step.

Instructor shall define grades for each point range earned upon completion of each performance-evaluated task.

Performance Standards

The minimum number of satisfactory performances required prior to final evaluation is _____.

Instructor shall identify by * those steps considered critical. If step is missed or minimum competency is not met, the evaluated procedure fails and must be repeated.

Performance Criteria	*	Self	Peer	Instructor	Comments
1. Loads the panoramic cassette in the darkroom under safelight conditions. Handles the film only by its edges to prevent fingerprints.					
2. Places all infection control barriers and containers.					
3. Covers the bite-block with a disposable plastic barrier. If the bite-block is not covered, it must be sterilized before used on the next patient.					
4. Covers or disinfects (or both) any part of the machine that comes in contact with the patient.					
5. Sets the exposure factors (kilovoltage, milliamperage) according to the manufacturer's recommendations.					
6. Adjusts the machine to accommodate the height of the patient; aligns all movable parts properly.					
7. Loads the cassette into the carrier of the panoramic unit.					

Additional Comments

Total number of points possible _____

Total number of points received _____

Grade _____ *Instructor's initials* _____ *Date* _____

177

COMPETENCY 17-14 PREPARING THE PATIENT FOR PANORAMIC RADIOGRAPHY

Performance Objective

By following a routine procedure that meets stated protocols, the student will be able to prepare a patient for panoramic radiography.

Evaluation and Grading Criteria

3	Student competently met the stated criteria without assistance.
2	Student required assistance in order to meet the stated criteria.
1	Student showed uncertainty when performing the stated criteria.
0	Student was not prepared and needs to repeat the step.
N/A	No evaluation of this step.

Instructor shall define grades for each point range earned upon completion of each performance-evaluated task.

Performance Standards

The minimum number of satisfactory performances required prior to final evaluation is _____.

Instructor shall identify by ∗ those steps considered critical. If step is missed or minimum competency is not met, the evaluated procedure fails and must be repeated.

Performance Criteria	∗	Self	Peer	Instructor	Comments
1. Explains procedure to the patient. Asks patient if he or she has any questions.					
2. Asks the patient to remove all objects from the head and neck area; this includes eyeglasses, earrings, lip-piercing and tongue-piercing objects, necklaces, napkin chains, hearing aids, hairpins, and complete and partial dentures. Places objects in a container.					
3. Places a double-sided lead apron on the patient or uses the style of lead apron recommended by the manufacturer.					

Additional Comments

Total number of points possible _____

Total number of points received _____

Grade _____ *Instructor's initials* _____ *Date* _____

179

Performance Objective

By following a routine procedure that meets stated protocols, the student will be able to position a patient for panoramic radiography.

Evaluation and Grading Criteria

3   Student competently met the stated criteria without assistance.

2   Student required assistance in order to meet the stated criteria.

1   Student showed uncertainty when performing the stated criteria.

0   Student was not prepared and needs to repeat the step.

N/A   No evaluation of this step.

Instructor shall define grades for each point range earned upon completion of each performance-evaluated task.

Performance Standards

The minimum number of satisfactory performances required prior to final evaluation is _____.

Instructor shall identify by * those steps considered critical. If step is missed or minimum competency is not met, the evaluated procedure fails and must be repeated.

Performance Criteria	*	Self	Peer	Instructor	Comments
1. Instructs the patient to sit or stand "as tall as possible" with his or her back straight and erect.					
2. Instructs the patient to bite on the plastic bite-block and then slide his or her upper and lower teeth into the notch (groove) on the end of the bite-block.					
3. Positions the mid-sagittal plane (the imaginary line that divides the patient's face into right and left sides) perpendicular to the floor.					
4. Positions the Frankfort plane (the imaginary plane that passes through the top of the ear canal and the bottom of the eye socket) parallel with the floor.					
5. Instructs the patient to position his or her tongue on the roof of the mouth and close his or her lips around the bite-block.					
6. After the patient has been positioned, instructs him or her to remain still while the machine rotates during exposure.					
7. Exposes the film and proceeds with film processing.					
8. Documents the procedure.					
Additional Comments					

Total number of points possible _____

Total number of points received _____

Grade _____ *Instructor's initials* _____ *Date* _____

18 Restorative and Esthetic Materials

TRUE/FALSE

_____ 1. Amalgam can also be referred to as an alloy.

_____ 2. IRM is the abbreviation for *intermediate resin matrix.*

_____ 3. Zinc Oxide-Eugenol is a versatile dental material that can be considered for use as a temporary cement, base, or permanent cement.

_____ 4. *Luting agent* is another term used for composite resins.

_____ 5. Trituration is the mechanical process by which mercury and alloy powder are mixed together.

_____ 6. Calcium hydroxide is a type of cavity liner.

_____ 7. Etchant is a liquid or gel substance applied to the enamel or dentin surface for a specified time when preparing the tooth surface for a bonding material.

_____ 8. A base is placed in the cavity preparation before placement of the permanent restoration.

_____ 9. Zinc phosphate cement undergoes an exothermic reaction during the spatulation process.

_____ 10. Tooth-whitening products are available in toothpaste, fluoride, floss, mouth rinses, and chewing gum.

MATCHING

Match the following restorative materials with their application.

_____ 11. Calcium hydroxide

_____ 12. Composite resin

_____ 13. Conditioner and/or etchant

_____ 14. Amalgam

_____ 15. Polycarboxylate cement

_____ 16. Bonding agent

_____ 17. Glass ionomer cement

_____ 18. Cavity varnish

A. Permanent alloy restorative material for posterior teeth

B. Liner placed to regenerate and protect the pulp

C. Luting agent used for metal and ceramic restorations

D. Material that prepares tooth structure for bonding

E. Permanent tooth colored restorative material

F. Material that seals dentinal tubules

G. Material that creates an adherence between the dental material and tooth structure

H. Luting agent for cast restoration and cementation of orthodontic bands

Match the properties of dental materials to their description.

_____ 19. Mechanical

_____ 20. Thermal

_____ 21. Electrical

_____ 22. Corrosive

_____ 23. Solubility

_____ 24. Application

A. The degree to which a substance will dissolve in a given amount of a wet environment

B. Reaction of the metal when it comes into contact with acidic products

C. Specific steps in placing the material

D. A current created by the interaction of metals with saliva

E. Temperature change in the mouth

F. Biting and chewing in the posterior area of the mouth

SHORT ANSWER

25. Provide the composition of amalgam.

COMPETENCY 18-1 MIXING AND TRANSFERRING DENTAL AMALGAM

Performance Objective

By following a routine procedure that meets stated protocols, the student will be able to mix and transfer dental amalgam.

Evaluation and Grading Criteria

3   Student competently met the stated criteria without assistance.

2   Student required assistance in order to meet the stated criteria.

1   Student showed uncertainty when performing the stated criteria.

0   Student was not prepared and needs to repeat the step.

N/A   No evaluation of this step.

Instructor shall define grades for each point range earned upon completion of each performance-evaluated task.

Performance Standards

The minimum number of satisfactory performances required prior to final evaluation is _____.

Instructor shall identify by ∗ those steps considered critical. If step is missed or minimum competency is not met, the evaluated procedure fails and must be repeated.

Performance Criteria	∗	Self	Peer	Instructor	Comments
1. Selects the proper equipment and supplies.					
2. Places personal protective equipment according to procedure.					
3. Prepares the amalgam capsule using the activator.					
4. Places the capsule in the amalgamator.					
5. Adjusts the settings on the amalgamator based on the type of amalgam.					
6. Closes the cover on the amalgamator and begins trituration.					
7. Removes the capsule, twists it open, and dispenses amalgam in the well or amalgam cloth.					
8. Fills both ends of the carrier.					
9. Transfers the carrier to the operator with the small end facing toward the tooth preparation.					
10. Continues this process until the preparation is overfilled.					

Additional Comments

Total number of points possible _____

Total number of points received _____

Grade _____ Instructor's initials _____ Date _____

185

COMPETENCY 18-2 PREPARING COMPOSITE RESIN MATERIALS

Performance Objective

By following a routine procedure that meets stated protocols, the student will be able to prepare composite resin materials.

Evaluation and Grading Criteria

3   Student competently met the stated criteria without assistance.

2   Student required assistance in order to meet the stated criteria.

1   Student showed uncertainty when performing the stated criteria.

0   Student was not prepared and needs to repeat the step.

N/A   No evaluation of this step.

Instructor shall define grades for each point range earned upon completion of each performance-evaluated task.

Performance Standards

The minimum number of satisfactory performances required prior to final evaluation is _____.

Instructor shall identify by ∗ those steps considered critical. If step is missed or minimum competency is not met, the evaluated procedure fails and must be repeated.

Performance Criteria	∗	Self	Peer	Instructor	Comments
1. Selects equipment and material.					
2. Places personal protective equipment according to procedure.					
3. Selects the shade of the tooth using a shade guide using natural lighting.					
4. Retrieves the composite resin syringe material and attaches a new tip to the syringe.					
5. Readies the etchant and bonding agent to be readied during placement of material.					
6. Transfers the composite syringe in the transfer zone to the dentist.					
7. Transfers the composite instrument in the transfer zone to the dentist.					
8. Readies the curing light during placement of the material. It is best when the material can be light-cured in increments.					

Additional Comments

Total number of points possible _____

Total number of points received _____

Grade _____ Instructor's initials _____ Date _____

COMPETENCY 18-3 APPLICATION OF CALCIUM HYDROXIDE (EXPANDED FUNCTION)

Performance Objective

By following a routine procedure that meets stated protocols, the student will assemble the necessary supplies and then will correctly manipulate and place the cavity liner in a prepared tooth.

Evaluation and Grading Criteria

3   Student competently met the stated criteria without assistance.

2   Student required assistance in order to meet the stated criteria.

1   Student showed uncertainty when performing the stated criteria.

0   Student was not prepared and needs to repeat the step.

N/A   No evaluation of this step.

Instructor shall define grades for each point range earned on completion of each performance-evaluated task.

Performance Standards

The minimum number of satisfactory performances required before final evaluation is _____.

Instructor shall identify by ∗ those steps considered critical. If step is missed or minimum competency is not met, the evaluated procedure fails and must be repeated.

Performance Criteria	∗	Self	Peer	Instructor	Comment
1. Selects the proper material and assembles the appropriate supplies.					
2. Places personal protective equipment according to procedure.					
3. Identifies preparation and where material is to be placed.					
4. Dispenses small, equal quantities of the catalyst and the base pastes onto the paper mixing pad.					
5. Uses a circular motion to mix the material over a small area of the paper pad with the spatula.					
6. Uses gauze to clean the spatula.					
7. With the tip of the applicator, picks up a small amount of the material and applies a thin layer at the deepest area of the preparation.					
8. Uses an explorer to remove any excess material from the enamel before drying.					

Performance Criteria	*	Self	Peer	Instructor	Comment
9. Cleans and disinfects the equipment.					
10. Procedure documented in patient record.					
Additional Comments					

Total number of points possible _____

Total number of points received _____

Grade _____ *Instructor's initials* _____ *Date* _____

COMPETENCY 18-4 APPLICATION OF DENTAL VARNISH (EXPANDED FUNCTION)

Performance Objective

By following a routine procedure that meets stated protocols, the student will assemble the necessary supplies and then will correctly apply dental varnish to a prepared tooth surface.

Evaluation and Grading Criteria

3   Student competently met the stated criteria without assistance.

2   Student required assistance in order to meet the stated criteria.

1   Student showed uncertainty when performing the stated criteria.

0   Student was not prepared and needs to repeat the step.

N/A   No evaluation of this step.

Instructor shall define grades for each point range earned on completion of each performance-evaluated task.

Performance Standards

The minimum number of satisfactory performances required before final evaluation is _____.

Instructor shall identify by * those steps considered critical. If step is missed or minimum competency is not met, the evaluated procedure fails and must be repeated.

Performance Criteria	*	Self	Peer	Instructor	Comment
1. Selects the proper material and assembles the appropriate supplies.					
2. Places personal protective equipment according to procedure.					
3. Identifies cavity preparation and where material is to be placed.					
4. Retrieves the applicator or sterile cotton pellets in cotton pliers.					
5. Opens the bottle of varnish and placed the tip of the applicator or cotton pellet into the liquid, making sure not to wet the cotton pliers.					
6. Replaces the cap on the bottle immediately.					
7. Places a coating of the varnish on the walls, floor, and margin of the cavity preparation.					
8. Applies a second coat.					

191

Performance Criteria	*	Self	Peer	Instructor	Comment
9. Cleans and disinfects the equipment.					
10. Procedure documented in patient record.					
Additional Comments					

Total number of points possible _____

Total number of points received _____

Grade _____ *Instructor's initials* _____ *Date* _____

Performance Objective

By following a routine procedure that meets stated protocols, the student will assemble the necessary supplies and then will correctly apply etchant to a prepared tooth surface.

Evaluation and Grading Criteria

3 Student competently met the stated criteria without assistance.

2 Student required assistance in order to meet the stated criteria.

1 Student showed uncertainty when performing the stated criteria.

0 Student was not prepared and needs to repeat the step.

N/A No evaluation of this step.

Instructor shall define grades for each point range earned on completion of each performance-evaluated task.

Performance Standards

The minimum number of satisfactory performances required before final evaluation is _____.

Instructor shall identify by * those steps considered critical. If step is missed or minimum competency is not met, the evaluated procedure fails and must be repeated.

Performance Criteria	*	Self	Peer	Instructor	Comment
1. Selects the proper material and assembles the appropriate supplies.					
2. Places personal protective equipment according to procedure.					
3. Identifies cavity outline and where material is placed.					
4. Uses a dental dam or cotton rolls to isolate the prepared tooth.					
5. Ensures that the surface of the tooth structure is clean and free of any debris, plaque, or calculus before etching.					
6. Carefully dries (but does not desiccate) the surface.					
7. Applies etchant to the enamel or dentin.					
8. Etches the tooth structure for the time recommended by the manufacturer.					
9. After etching, thoroughly rinses and dries the surface for 15-30 seconds.					
10. Ensures that the etched surface has a frosty-white appearance.					

Performance Criteria	*	Self	Peer	Instructor	Comment
11. When finished, cares for supplies and materials appropriately.					
12. Documents procedure in patient record.					
Additional Comments					

Total number of points possible _____

Total number of points received _____

Grade _____ *Instructor's initials* _____ *Date* _____

COMPETENCY 18-6 APPLYING A BONDING SYSTEM (EXPANDED FUNCTION)

Performance Objective

By following a routine procedure that meets stated protocols, the student will assemble the necessary supplies and then will correctly apply a bonding system to a prepared tooth surface.

Evaluation and Grading Criteria

3   Student competently met the stated criteria without assistance.

2   Student required assistance in order to meet the stated criteria.

1   Student showed uncertainty when performing the stated criteria.

0   Student was not prepared and needs to repeat the step.

N/A   No evaluation of this step.

Instructor shall define grades for each point range earned on completion of each performance-evaluated task.

Performance Standards

The minimum number of satisfactory performances required before final evaluation is _____.

Instructor shall identify by * those steps considered critical. If step is missed or minimum competency is not met, the evaluated procedure fails and must be repeated.

Performance Criteria	*	Self	Peer	Instructor	Comment
1. Selects the proper material and assembles the appropriate supplies.					
2. Places personal protective equipment according to procedure.					
3. Identifies cavity outline and placement of material.					
4. If a metal matrix band is required, prepares the band with cavity varnish or wax before placement around the tooth.					
5. Etches the cavity preparation and the enamel margins according to the manufacturer's instructions.					
6. If a primer is part of the system, applies a primer to the entire preparation in one or multiple coats, depending on the manufacturer's instructions.					
7. Places the dual-cured bonding resin in the entire cavity preparation and lightly air-thins the material. The resin should appear unset or semiset.					
8. When finished, cares for supplies and materials appropriately.					
9. Documents procedure in patient record.					
Additional Comments					

Total number of points possible _____

Total number of points received _____

Grade _____ *Instructor's initials* _____ *Date* _____

195

Performance Objective

By following a routine procedure that meets stated protocols, the student will be able to mix intermediate restorative materials.

Evaluation and Grading Criteria

3   Student competently met the stated criteria without assistance.

2   Student required assistance in order to meet the stated criteria.

1   Student showed uncertainty when performing the stated criteria.

0   Student was not prepared and needs to repeat the step.

N/A   No evaluation of this step.

Instructor shall define grades for each point range earned upon completion of each performance-evaluated task.

Performance Standards

The minimum number of satisfactory performances required prior to final evaluation is _____.

Instructor shall identify by * those steps considered critical. If step is missed or minimum competency is not met, the evaluated procedure fails and must be repeated.

Performance Criteria	*	Self	Peer	Instructor	Comments
1. Selects the proper material and assembles the appropriate supplies.					
2. Places personal protective equipment according to procedure.					
3. Shakes the powder bottle before dispensing; then measures the powder onto the mixing pad. Recaps the bottle.					
4. Makes a well in half the powder; dispenses the liquid into the well. Recaps the bottle.					
5. Incorporates the remaining powder into the mixture in two or three increments, and mixes thoroughly with the spatula. The mix is quite stiff at this stage.					
6. Wipes the mix back and forth on the mixing pad for 5–10 seconds. The resulting mix should be smooth and adaptable.					
7. Completes the mix within 1 minute. Readies the material in one mass.					
8. Cleans and disinfects the equipment immediately.					
Additional Comments					

Total number of points possible _____

Total number of points received _____

Grade _____ *Instructor's initials* _____ *Date* _____

COMPETENCY 18-8 MIXING GLASS IONOMER FOR PERMANENT CEMENTATION

Performance Objective

By following a routine procedure that meets stated protocols, the student will assemble the necessary supplies and will correctly manipulate the material for use in the cementation of a cast crown.

Evaluation and Grading Criteria

3   Student competently met the stated criteria without assistance.

2   Student required assistance in order to meet the stated criteria.

1   Student showed uncertainty when performing the stated criteria.

0   Student was not prepared and needs to repeat the step.

N/A   No evaluation of this step.

Instructor shall define grades for each point range earned on completion of each performance-evaluated task.

Performance Standards

The minimum number of satisfactory performances required before final evaluation is _____.

Instructor shall identify by * those steps considered critical. If step is missed or minimum competency is not met, the evaluated procedure fails and must be repeated.

Performance Criteria	*	Self	Peer	Instructor	Comment
1. Selects the proper material and assembles the appropriate supplies.					
2. Places personal protective equipment according to procedure.					
3. Dispenses the manufacturer's recommended proportion of the *liquid* on one half of the paper pad.					
4. Dispenses the manufacturer's recommended proportion of the *powder* on the other half of the pad; this usually is divided into two or three increments.					
5. Incorporates the powder into the liquid for the recommended mixing time until the material has a glossy appearance.					
6. Lines inside of crown with cement.					
7. Turns the casting over in the palm and transfers it to the dentist.					
8. Transfers a cotton roll so the patient can bite down on it to help seat the crown and displace the excess cement.					
9. When finished, cares for supplies and materials appropriately.					

Additional Comments

Total number of points possible _____

Total number of points received _____

Grade _____ Instructor's initials _____ Date _____

COMPETENCY 18-9 MIXING COMPOSITE RESIN FOR PERMANENT CEMENTATION

Performance Objective

By following a routine procedure that meets stated protocols, the student will assemble the necessary supplies and will correctly manipulate the material for use in the cementation of a cast crown.

Evaluation and Grading Criteria

3	Student competently met the stated criteria without assistance.
2	Student required assistance in order to meet the stated criteria.
1	Student showed uncertainty when performing the stated criteria.
0	Student was not prepared and needs to repeat the step.
N/A	No evaluation of this step.

Instructor shall define grades for each point range earned on completion of each performance-evaluated task.

Performance Standards

The minimum number of satisfactory performances required before final evaluation is _____.

Instructor shall identify by * those steps considered critical. If step is missed or minimum competency is not met, the evaluated procedure fails and must be repeated.

Performance Criteria	*	Self	Peer	Instructor	Comment
1. Selected the proper material and assembled the appropriate supplies.					
2. Placed personal protective equipment according to procedure.					
3. Applied etchant to enamel and dentin for 15 seconds and then rinsed. Blotted excess water with a moist cotton pellet, leaving the tooth moist.					
4. Applied a bond adhesive to the enamel and dentin and dried gently. Avoided excess adhesive on all prepared surfaces.					
5. Light-cured each surface for 10 seconds.					
6. Applied primer to etched porcelain or roughened metal surfaces. Dried for 5 seconds.					
7. Dispensed a 1:1 ratio of powder to liquid onto a mixing pad and mixed for 10 seconds. Applied a thin layer of cement to the bonding surface of the restoration.					
8. After the crown was seated, light-cured the margins for 40 seconds or allowed to self-cure for 10 minutes from the start of the mixing.					
9. When finished, cared for supplies and materials appropriately.					

Additional Comments

201

COMPETENCY 18-10 MIXING ZINC OXIDE–EUGENOL FOR A BASE, TEMPORARY CEMENTATION, AND PERMANENT CEMENTATION

Performance Objective

By following a routine procedure that meets stated protocols, the student will assemble the necessary supplies and will correctly manipulate ZOE for permanent cementation.

Evaluation and Grading Criteria

3   Student competently met the stated criteria without assistance.

2   Student required assistance in order to meet the stated criteria.

1   Student showed uncertainty when performing the stated criteria.

0   Student was not prepared and needs to repeat the step.

N/A   No evaluation of this step.

Instructor shall define grades for each point range earned on completion of each performance-evaluated task.

Performance Standards

The minimum number of satisfactory performances required before final evaluation is _____.

Instructor shall identify by ∗ those steps considered critical. If step is missed or minimum competency is not met, the evaluated procedure fails and must be repeated.

Performance Criteria	∗	Self	Peer	Instructor	Comment
ZOE as a Base					
1. Measures the powder onto the mixing pad. Replaces cap immediately.					
2. Dispenses the liquid near the powder on the mixing pad. Replaces the cap on the liquid container immediately.					
3. Incorporates half the powder into the liquid; mixes with the spatula for 20–30 seconds.					
4. Incorporates the remaining portion into the mixture. Continues mixing for an additional 20–30 seconds. The material should be thick and putty-like.					
ZOE as Permanent Cement					
1. Measures the powder and places it onto the mixing pad. Replaces the cap on the powder immediately.					
2. Dispenses the liquid near the powder on the mixing pad. Replaces the cap on the liquid container immediately.					
3. Incorporates the powder and liquid all at once, and mixes them with the spatula for 30 seconds.					
4. After ensuring a putty-like consistency of the initial mix, mixes for an additional 30 seconds until it becomes more fluid for loading into a casting.					

Performance Criteria	*	Self	Peer	Instructor	Comment
5. Lines the crown with the permanent cement.					
6. Inverts crown in the palm and readies for transfer.					
Additional Comments					

Total number of points possible _____

Total number of points received _____

Grade _____ Instructor's initials _____ Date _____

COMPETENCY 18-11: MIXING POLYCARBOXYLATE FOR A BASE AND PERMANENT CEMENTATION

Performance Objective

By following a routine procedure that meets stated protocols, the student will assemble the necessary supplies and will correctly manipulate the material for use in cementation.

Evaluation and Grading Criteria

3   Student competently met the stated criteria without assistance.

2   Student required assistance in order to meet the stated criteria.

1   Student showed uncertainty when performing the stated criteria.

0   Student was not prepared and needs to repeat the step.

N/A   No evaluation of this step.

Instructor shall define grades for each point range earned on completion of each performance-evaluated task.

Performance Standards

The minimum number of satisfactory performances required before final evaluation is _____.

Instructor shall identify by * those steps considered critical. If step is missed or minimum competency is not met, the evaluated procedure fails and must be repeated.

Performance Criteria	*	Self	Peer	Instructor	Comment
Polycarboxylate for a Base					
1. Dispenses the powder and liquid onto the pad.					
2. Incorporates all the powder into the liquid, with total mixing time not to exceed 45 seconds.					
3. Forms the completed mix into a small ball.					
Polycarboxylate for Permanent Cement					
1. Gently shakes the powder to fluff the ingredients.					
2. Measures the powder onto the mixing pad and immediately recaps the container.					
3. Dispenses the liquid and then recaps the container.					
4. Uses the flat side of the spatula to incorporate all the powder quickly into the liquid at one time. The mix is completed within 30 seconds.					
5. Ensures that the mix is somewhat thick with a shiny, glossy surface.					
6. Lines inside of crown with cement.					
7. Turns the casting over in the palm and transfers it to the dentist.					
8. Transfers a cotton roll so the patient can bite down on it to help seat the crown and displace the excess cement.					
9. When finished, cares for supplies and materials appropriately.					

Performance Criteria	*	Self	Peer	Instructor	Comment
Additional Comments					

Total number of points possible _____

Total number of points received _____

Grade _____ *Instructor's initials* _____ *Date* _____

COMPETENCY 18-12 MIXING ZINC PHOSPHATE FOR A BASE AND PERMANENT CEMENTATION

Performance Objective

By following a routine procedure that meets stated protocols, the student will assemble the necessary supplies and will correctly manipulate the material for use in the cementation of a cast crown.

Evaluation and Grading Criteria

3   Student competently met the stated criteria without assistance.

2   Student required assistance in order to meet the stated criteria.

1   Student showed uncertainty when performing the stated criteria.

0   Student was not prepared and needs to repeat the step.

N/A   No evaluation of this step.

Instructor shall define grades for each point range earned on completion of each performance-evaluated task.

Performance Standards

The minimum number of satisfactory performances required before final evaluation is _____.

Instructor shall identify by * those steps considered critical. If step is missed or minimum competency is not met, the evaluated procedure fails and must be repeated.

Performance Criteria	*	Self	Peer	Instructor	Comment
Zinc Phosphate for a Base					
1. Dispenses the powder and liquid onto the pad.					
2. Incorporates all the powder into the liquid, with total mixing time not to exceed 45 seconds.					
3. Forms the completed mix into a small ball.					
Zinc Phosphate for Permanent Cementation: Preparing the Mix					
1. Cools and dries glass slab for mixing.					
2. Dispenses the powder toward one end of the slab and the liquid at the opposite end. Recaps the containers.					
3. Divides the powder into small increments as directed by the manufacturer.					
4. Incorporates each powder increment into the liquid, beginning with smaller increments.					
5. Spatulates the mix thoroughly, using broad strokes or a figure-eight movement over a large area of the slab.					
6. Tests the material for appropriate cementation consistency. (The cement should string up and break about 1 inch from the slab.)					

207

Performance Criteria	*	Self	Peer	Instructor	Comment
Placing Cement in the Casting					
1. Holds the casting with the inner portion facing upward.					
2. Retrieves the cement onto the spatula. Scrapes the edge of the spatula along the margin to cause the cement to flow from the spatula into the casting.					
3. Places the tip of the spatula or a black spoon into the bulk of the cement and moves the material so that it covers all internal walls with a thin lining of cement.					
4. Turns the casting over in the palm and transfers it to the dentist.					
5. Transfers a cotton roll so the patient can bite down on it to help seat the crown and displace the excess cement.					
6. When finished, cares for supplies and materials appropriately.					
Additional Comments					

Total number of points possible _____

Total number of points received _____

Grade _____ *Instructor's initials* _____ *Date* _____

19 Impression Materials and Laboratory Procedures

TRUE/FALSE

_____ 1. A quadrant impression tray covers half of a dental arch.

_____ 2. When an impression is poured in stone, you are creating a negative reproduction of the teeth and the surrounding structures.

_____ 3. Alginate is an irreversible hydrocolloid.

_____ 4. The water-to-powder ratio for mixing alginate for the maxillary tray is one scoop of powder to the second "measure line" of water.

_____ 5. A *diagnostic cast* is the model that is fabricated from the impression.

_____ 6. Dental stone is a weaker material than model plaster.

_____ 7. The dental cast is trimmed using a laboratory handpiece.

_____ 8. When taking a final impression, the heavy body material is placed in the tray.

_____ 9. Another term for occlusal registration is *bite registration.*

_____ 10. The two most common ways to mix final impression materials are mixing two pastes or the use of an amalgamator.

MATCHING

Match the type of impression material with its use (answer choices can be used more than once).

_____ 11. Alginate   A. Preliminary impression

_____ 12. Polysulfide   B. Final impression

_____ 13. Wax   C. Occlusal registration

_____ 14. Condensation silicone

_____ 15. Polyether

SHORT ANSWER

16. List the five factors that influence the setting of gypsum.

17. List two types of impression trays and describe their characteristics.

Performance Objective

By following a routine procedure that meets stated protocols, the student will mix alginate impression material.

Evaluation and Grading Criteria

3   Student competently met the stated criteria without assistance.

2   Student required assistance in order to meet the stated criteria.

1   Student showed uncertainty when performing the stated criteria.

0   Student was not prepared and needs to repeat the step.

N/A   No evaluation of this step.

Instructor shall define grades for each point range earned on completion of each performance-evaluated task.

Performance Standards

The minimum number of satisfactory performances required before final evaluation is _____.

Instructor shall identify by * those steps considered critical. If step is missed or minimum competency is not met, the evaluated procedure fails and must be repeated.

Performance Criteria	*	Self	Peer	Instructor	Comment
1. Gathers appropriate supplies.					
2. Places personal protective equipment according to procedure.					
3. Places the appropriate amount of water into the bowl using the calibrated measure.					
4. Shakes the can of alginate to "fluff" the contents. After fluffing, carefully lifts the lid to prevent the particles from flying into the air.					
5. Using the correct scoop, sifts the powder into the water.					
6. Uses the spatula to mix with a stirring action to wet the powder until it is all moistened.					
7. Firmly spreads the alginate between the spatula and the side of the rubber bowl.					
8. Spatulates material for the appropriate length of time, until the mixture appears smooth and creamy.					
9. Wipes the alginate mix into one mass on the inside edge of the bowl.					
10. When finished, cares for supplies and materials appropriately.					
Additional Comments					

Total number of points possible _____

Total number of points received _____

Grade _____ *Instructor's initials* _____ *Date* _____

COMPETENCIES 19-2 AND 19-3 TAKING A MANDIBULAR AND MAXILLARY PRELIMINARY IMPRESSION (EXPANDED FUNCTION)

Performance Objective

By following a routine procedure that meets stated protocols, the student will take a mandibular and maxillary alginate impression of diagnostic quality.

Evaluation and Grading Criteria

3   Student competently met the stated criteria without assistance.

2   Student required assistance in order to meet the stated criteria.

1   Student showed uncertainty when performing the stated criteria.

0   Student was not prepared and needs to repeat the step.

N/A   No evaluation of this step.

Instructor shall define grades for each point range earned on completion of each performance-evaluated task.

Performance Standards

The minimum number of satisfactory performances required before final evaluation is _____.

Instructor shall identify by * those steps considered critical. If step is missed or minimum competency is not met, the evaluated procedure fails and must be repeated.

Performance Criteria	*	Self	Peer	Instructor	Comment
1. Gathers all necessary supplies.					
2. Places personal protective equipment according to procedure.					
3. Seats and prepares the patient.					
4. Explains the procedure to the patient.					
Taking the Mandibular Impression					
1. Selects and prepares the mandibular impression tray.					
2. Obtains two measures of room-temperature water with two scoops of alginate and mixes the material.					
3. Gathers half the alginate in the bowl onto the spatula, then wipes alginate into one side of the tray from the lingual side. Quickly presses the material down to the base of the tray.					
4. Gathers the remaining half of the alginate in the bowl onto the spatula and then loads the other side of the tray in the same way.					
5. Smooths the surface of the alginate by wiping a moistened finger along the surface.					
6. Places additional material over the occlusal surfaces of the mandibular teeth.					
7. Retracts the patient's cheek with the index finger.					
8. Turns the tray slightly sideways when placing it into the mouth.					

213

Performance Criteria	*	Self	Peer	Instructor	Comment
9. Centers the tray over the teeth.					
10. Seats the tray from the posterior border first.					
11. Instructs the patient to breathe normally while the material set.					
12. Observes the alginate around the tray to determine when the material had set.					
13. Places fingers on top of the impression tray and gently breaks the seal between the impression and the peripheral tissues by moving the inside of the patient's cheeks or lips with the finger.					
14. Grasps the handle of the tray with the thumb and index finger and uses a firm lifting motion to break the seal.					
15. Snaps up the tray and impression from the dentition.					
16. Instructs the patient to rinse with water to remove excess alginate material.					
17. Evaluates the impression for accuracy.					
18. Procedure documented in patient record.					
Taking the Maxillary Impression **Loading the Maxillary Impression Tray**					
1. For a maxillary impression, mixes three measures of water and three scoops of powder.					
2. Loads the maxillary tray in one large increment and uses a wiping motion to fill the tray from the posterior end.					
3. Places the bulk of the material toward the anterior palatal area of the tray.					
4. Moistens fingertips with tap water and smooths the surface of the alginate.					
5. Uses the index finger to retract the patient's cheek.					
6. Turns the tray slightly sideways to position the tray into the mouth.					
7. Centers the tray over the patient's teeth.					
8. Seats the posterior border (back) of the tray up against the posterior border of the hard palate to form a seal.					
9. Directs the anterior portion of the tray upward over the teeth.					
10. Gently lifts the patient's lips out of the way as the tray is seated and instructs the patient to tilt head forward.					
11. Checks the posterior border of the tray to ensure that no material is flowing into the patient's throat. If necessary, wipes excess material away with a cotton-tipped applicator.					
12. Holds the tray firmly in place while the alginate sets.					

Performance Criteria	*	Self	Peer	Instructor	Comment
13. To avoid injury to the impression and the patient's teeth, places a finger along the lateral borders of the tray to push down and break the palatal seal.					
14. Uses a straight, downward snapping motion to remove the tray from the teeth.					
15. Instructs the patient to rinse with water to remove any excess alginate impression material.					
16. Gently rinses the impression under cold tap water to remove any blood or saliva.					
17. Sprays the impression with an approved disinfectant.					
18. Wraps the impression in a damp paper towel and stores it in a covered container or a plastic biohazard bag labeled with the patient's name.					
19. Examines the patient's mouth for any remaining fragments of alginate and removes them using an explorer and dental floss.					
20. Uses a moist facial tissue to remove any alginate from the patient's face and lips.					
21. Procedure documented in patient record.					
Additional Comments					

Total number of points possible _____

Total number of points received _____

Grade _____ *Instructor's initials* _____ *Date* _____

Performance Objective

By following a routine procedure that meets stated protocols, the student will prepare and mix a two-paste final impression material.

Evaluation and Grading Criteria

3	Student competently met the stated criteria without assistance.
2	Student required assistance in order to meet the stated criteria.
1	Student showed uncertainty when performing the stated criteria.
0	Student was not prepared and needs to repeat the step.
N/A	No evaluation of this step.

Instructor shall define grades for each point range earned on completion of each performance-evaluated task.

Performance Standards

The minimum number of satisfactory performances required before final evaluation is _____.

Instructor shall identify by * those steps considered critical. If step is missed or minimum competency is not met, the evaluated procedure fails and must be repeated.

Performance Criteria	*	Self	Peer	Instructor	Comment
1. Gathers appropriate supplies.					
2. Places personal protective equipment according to procedure.					
Preparing Light-Bodied Syringe Material					
1. Dispenses approximately 1½ to 2 inches of equal lengths of the base and catalyst of the light-bodied material onto the top third of the pad, ensuring that the materials are not too close to each other.					
2. Wipes the tube openings clean with gauze and recaps immediately.					
3. Places the tip of the spatula blade into the catalyst and base and mixes in a swirling direction for approximately 5 seconds.					
4. Gathers the material onto the flat portion of the spatula and places it on a clean area of the pad, preferably the center.					
5. Spatulates smoothly, wiping back and forth, and trying to use only one side of the spatula during the mixing process.					
6. To obtain a more homogenous mix, picks the material up by the spatula blade and wipes it onto the pad.					
7. Gathers the material together, takes the syringe tube, and begins "cookie cutting" the material into the syringe. Inserts the plunger and expresses a small amount of the material to ensure that the syringe is in working order.					
8. Transfers the syringe to the dentist, ensuring that the tip of the syringe is directed toward the tooth.					

Performance Criteria	*	Self	Peer	Instructor	Comment
Preparing Heavy-Bodied Tray Material					
1. Dispenses equal lengths of the base and catalyst of the heavy-bodied material on the top third of the pad for a quadrant tray.					
2. Places the tip of the spatula blade into the catalyst and base and mixes in a swirling direction for approximately 5 seconds.					
3. Gathers the material onto the flat portion of the spatula, and places it onto a clean area of the pad.					
4. Spatulates smoothly, wiping back and forth using only one side of the spatula during the mixing process.					
5. To get a more homogenous mix, picks the material up with the spatula blade and wipes it onto the pad.					
6. Gathers the bulk of the material with the spatula and loads the material into the tray.					
7. Using the tip of the spatula, spreads the material evenly from one end of the tray to the other without picking up the material.					
8. Retrieves the syringe from the dentist and transfers the tray, ensuring that the dentist can grasp the handle of the tray properly.					
9. When finished, cares for supplies and materials appropriately.					
10. Documents procedure in patient record.					
Additional Comments					

Total number of points possible _____

Total number of points received _____

Grade _____ *Instructor's initials* _____ *Date* _____

COMPETENCY 19-5 PREPARING AN AUTOMIX FINAL IMPRESSION MATERIAL

Performance Objective

By following a routine procedure that meets stated protocols, the student will prepare an automix final impression material.

Evaluation and Grading Criteria

3   Student competently met the stated criteria without assistance.

2   Student required assistance in order to meet the stated criteria.

1   Student showed uncertainty when performing the stated criteria.

0   Student was not prepared and needs to repeat the step.

N/A   No evaluation of this step.

Instructor shall define grades for each point range earned on completion of each performance-evaluated task.

Performance Standards

The minimum number of satisfactory performances required before final evaluation is _____.

Instructor shall identify by * those steps considered critical. If step is missed or minimum competency is not met, the evaluated procedure fails and must be repeated.

Performance Criteria	*	Self	Peer	Instructor	Comment
1. Gathers appropriate supplies.					
2. Places personal protective equipment according to procedure.					
3. Loads the extruder with dual cartridges of the base and the catalyst of light-bodied material.					
4. Removes the caps from the tube and extrudes a small amount of unmixed material onto the gauze pad.					
5. Attaches a mixing tip on the extruder along with a syringe tip for light-bodied application by the dentist.					
6. When the dentist signals, begins squeezing the trigger until the material reaches the tip.					
7. Transfers the extruder to the dentist, directing the tip toward the area of the impression.					
8. Places the heavy-bodied cartridges in the extruder, expressing a small amount as before with the light-bodied material. Attaches the mixing tip to the cartridge.					
9. When the dentist signals, begins squeezing the trigger, mixing the heavy-bodied material.					
10. Loads the impression tray with heavy-bodied material, making sure not to trap air in the material.					
11. Transfers the tray, ensuring that the dentist can grasp the handle of the tray.					

219

Performance Criteria	*	Self	Peer	Instructor	Comment
12. Disinfects the impression, places it in a biohazard bag, labels it with the patient's name, and readies it for the laboratory.					
13. Documents procedure in patient record.					
Additional Comments					

Total number of points possible _____

Total number of points received _____

Grade _____ Instructor's initials _____ Date _____

Performance Objective

By following a routine procedure that meets stated protocols, the student will be able to mix dental plaster.

Evaluation and Grading Criteria

3   Student competently met the stated criteria without assistance.

2   Student required assistance in order to meet the stated criteria.

1   Student showed uncertainty when performing the stated criteria.

0   Student was not prepared and needs to repeat the step.

N/A   No evaluation of this step.

Instructor shall define grades for each point range earned upon completion of each performance-evaluated task.

Performance Standards

The minimum number of satisfactory performances required prior to final evaluation is _____.

Instructor shall identify by * those steps considered critical. If step is missed or minimum competency is not met, the evaluated procedure fails and must be repeated.

Performance Criteria	*	Self	Peer	Instructor	Comments
1. Gathers appropriate supplies.					
2. Places personal protective equipment according to procedure.					
3. Measures 50 mL of room-temperature water into a clean rubber mixing bowl.					
4. Places the paper towel on the scale and makes necessary adjustments.					
5. Weighs out 100 g of dental plaster.					
6. Adds the powder to the water in steady increment. Allows the powder to settle into the water for approximately 30 seconds.					
7. Uses the spatula to incorporate the powder slowly into the water. A smooth and creamy mix should be achieved in about 20 seconds.					
8. Turns the vibrator to low or medium speed and places the bowl of plaster mix on the vibrator platform.					
9. Lightly presses and rotates the bowl on the vibrator, allowing air bubbles to rise to the surface.					
10. Completes mixing and vibration of the plaster within 2 minutes.					
Additional Comments					

Total number of points possible _____

Total number of points received _____

Grade _____ *Instructor's initials* _____ *Date* _____

Performance Objective

By following a routine procedure that meets stated protocols, the student will be able to pour dental models using the inverted-pour method.

Evaluation and Grading Criteria

3	Student competently met the stated criteria without assistance.
2	Student required assistance in order to meet the stated criteria.
1	Student showed uncertainty when performing the stated criteria.
0	Student was not prepared and needs to repeat the step.
N/A	No evaluation of this step.

Instructor shall define grades for each point range earned upon completion of each performance-evaluated task.

Performance Standards

The minimum number of satisfactory performances required prior to final evaluation is _____.

Instructor shall identify by * those steps considered critical. If step is missed or minimum competency is not met, the evaluated procedure fails and must be repeated.

Performance Criteria	*	Self	Peer	Instructor	Comments
1. Gathers the appropriate supplies.					
2. Places personal protective equipment according to procedure.					
Preparing the Impression					
1. Uses a gentle stream of air to remove excess moisture from the impression. Is careful not to dry out the impression.					
2. Uses a laboratory knife or laboratory cutters to remove any excess impression material that would interfere with the pouring of the model.					
Pouring the Mandibular Model and Base					
1. Mixes the plaster; then sets the vibrator at low to medium speed.					
2. Holds the impression tray by the handle and places the edge of the base of the handle on the vibrator.					
3. Dips the spatula into the plaster mix, picking up a small increment (about ½ tsp).					
4. Places that small increment in the impression near the most posterior tooth. Guides the material as it flows lingually.					
5. Continues to place small increments in the same area as the first increment and allows the plaster to flow toward the anterior teeth.					
6. Turns the tray on its side to provide continuous flow of material into each tooth impression.					

Performance Criteria	*	Self	Peer	Instructor	Comments
7. Once all of the teeth in the impression are covered, begins to add larger increments until the entire impression is filled.					
8. Places the additional material onto a glass slab (or tile); shapes the base to approximately 2 × 2 inches by 1 inch thick.					
9. Inverts the impression onto the new mix. Does not push the impression into the base.					
10. Holds the tray steady, using a spatula to smooth the plaster base mix up onto the margins of the initial pour. Is careful not to cover the impression tray with material.					
Pouring the Maxillary Cast					
1. Repeats steps 3 through 5 from "Pouring the Mandibular Model and Base," using clean equipment for the fresh mix of plaster.					
2. Places the small increment of plaster in the posterior area of the impression. Guides the material as it flows into the impression of the most posterior tooth.					
3. Continues to place small increments in the same area as the first increment and allows the plaster to flow toward the anterior teeth.					
4. Rotates the tray on its side to permit the continuous flow of material into each tooth impression.					
5. Once all the teeth in the impression are covered, begins to add larger increments until the entire impression is filled.					
6. Places the mix onto a glass slab (or tile) and shapes the base to approximately 2 × 2 inches by 1 inch thick.					
7. Inverts the impression onto the new mix. Does not push the impression into the base.					
8. Holding the tray steady, uses a spatula to smooth the stone base mix onto the margins of the initial pour. Is careful not to cover the impression tray with plaster.					
9. Places the impression tray on the base so that the handle and the occlusal plane of the teeth on the cast are parallel with the surface of the glass slab (or tile).					
Separating the Cast from the Impression					
1. Waits 45–60 minutes after the base has been poured before separating the impression from the model.					
2. Uses the laboratory knife to gently separate the margins of the tray.					
3. Applies a firm, straight, and upward pressure on the handle of the tray to remove the impression.					

Performance Criteria	*	Self	Peer	Instructor	Comments
4. If the tray does not separate easily, checks to see where the tray is still attached to the impression. Again, uses the laboratory knife to free the tray from the model.					
5. Pulls the tray handle straight up from the model.					
6. Readies the models for trimming and polishing.					
Additional Comments					

Total number of points possible _____

Total number of points received _____

Grade _____ *Instructor's initials* _____ *Date* _____

Chapter **19** **Impression Materials and Laboratory Procedures**

Performance Objective

By following a routine procedure that meets stated protocols, the student will be able to trim and finish dental models.

Evaluation and Grading Criteria

3   Student competently met the stated criteria without assistance.

2   Student required assistance in order to meet the stated criteria.

1   Student showed uncertainty when performing the stated criteria.

0   Student was not prepared and needs to repeat the step.

N/A   No evaluation of this step.

Instructor shall define grades for each point range earned upon completion of each performance-evaluated task.

Performance Standards

The minimum number of satisfactory performances required prior to final evaluation is _____.

Instructor shall identify by * those steps considered critical. If step is missed or minimum competency is not met, the evaluated procedure fails and must be repeated.

Performance Criteria	*	Self	Peer	Instructor	Comments
1. Gathers appropriate supplies.					
2. Places personal protective equipment according to procedure.					
Preparing the Model					
1. Soaks the art portion of the model in a bowl of water for a minimum of 5 minutes.					
Trimming the Maxillary Model					
1. Places the maxillary model on a flat countertop with the teeth setting on the table. Uses a pencil to measure up ¼ inch from the counter and draws a line around the model.					
2. Turns on the trimmer, holds the model firmly against the trimmer, and trims the bottom of the base to the line that was drawn.					
3. Draws a line ¼ inch behind the maxillary tuberosities. With the base flat on the trimmer, removes excess plaster in the posterior area of the model to the marked line.					
4. To trim the sides of the model draws a line through the center of the occlusal ridges on one side of the model. Measures out ¼ inch from this line and draws a line parallel to the previous line drawn.					
5. Repeats these measurements on the other side of the model.					
6. Trims the sides of the cast to the lines drawn.					
7. Draws a line behind the tuberosity that is perpendicular to the opposite canine and trims to that line. This completes the maxillary heel cuts.					

227

Chapter **19**   **Impression Materials and Laboratory Procedures**

Performance Criteria	*	Self	Peer	Instructor	Comments
8. The final cut is made from drawing a line from the canine to the midline at an angle. Completes this on both sides and trims to the line.					
Trimming the Mandibular Model					
1. Occludes the mandibular model with the maxillary model using the wax bite.					
2. With the mandibular base on the trimmer, trims the posterior portion of the mandibular model until it is even with the maxillary model.					
3. Places the models upside down (maxillary base on the table), measures 3 inches from the surface up, and marks a line around the base of the mandibular model.					
4. Trims the mandibular model base to the line drawn.					
5. With the models in occlusion with the wax bite, places the mandibular model on the trimmer and trims the lateral cuts to match the maxillary lateral cuts.					
6. Trims the back and heel cuts so that they are even with the maxillary heel cuts.					
7. Checks that the mandibular anterior cut is rounded from the mandibular right canine to the mandibular left canine.					
8. The models are ready for finishing.					
Finishing the Model					
1. Mixes a slurry of gypsum and water and fills in any voids.					
2. Using a laboratory knife, removes any extra gypsum that occurs as beads on the occlusion model.					
Additional Comments					

Total number of points possible _____

Total number of points received _____

Grade _____ *Instructor's initials* _____ *Date* _____

20 Preventive Care

TRUE/FALSE

_____ 1. Fluoridated drinking water contains approximately 0.7 mg/L of fluoride.

_____ 2. Fluoride is a naturally occurring mineral.

_____ 3. Flossing is most effective for occlusal surfaces of the teeth.

_____ 4. Disclosing agents are useful as teaching aids.

_____ 5. An oral health program is based on motivation and education.

FILL IN THE BLANK

Select the best term:
  Active Learning
  Bass
  Cariogenic
  Demineralization
  Dental Floss
  Fluorosis
  Interdental aids
  Remineralization
  Systemic
  Topical

6. _____ is caused by excessive amounts of fluoride.

7. _____ fluorides are also known as dietary fluorides.

8. _____ fluoride can be applied through the following methods: toothpaste, rinses, and gels.

9. _____ is the process by which decay begins.

10. _____ is the most effective way to learn.

11. A food that is _____ has the ability to cause dental decay.

12. _____ is used to remove plaque from interproximal surfaces.

13. _____ are used to clean large spaces between the teeth.

14. _____ is the process by which decay is stopped.

15. The most commonly recommended method of toothbrushing is the _____ technique.

MULTIPLE CHOICE

16. Which of the following is an effective interdental aid?
    a. interproximal brushes
    b. dental floss
    c. rubber and wooden-tip stimulators
    d. all of the above

17. Which is a common source of systemic fluoride?
    a. toothpaste
    b. mouth rinses
    c. fluoridated water
    d. all of the above

18. Which of the following would make a patient high risk for dental decay?
    a. having already had dental decay
    b. living in an area without public water fluoridation
    c. having a limited amount of saliva
    d. all of the above

19. Which of the following foods is the most cariogenic?
    a. sweet, sticky foods
    b. soft drinks
    c. fruits
    d. vegetables

20. Oral health education does not include:
    a. open communication
    b. listening to the patient's concerns
    c. providing reinforcement
    d. lecturing to the patient

Performance Objective

By following a routine procedure that meets stated protocols, the student will be able to assist a patient with dental floss.

Evaluation and Grading Criteria

3   Student competently met the stated criteria without assistance.

2   Student required assistance in order to meet the stated criteria.

1   Student showed uncertainty when performing the stated criteria.

0   Student was not prepared and needs to repeat the step.

N/A   No evaluation of this step.

Instructor shall define grades for each point range earned upon completion of each performance-evaluated task.

Performance Standards

The minimum number of satisfactory performances required prior to final evaluation is _____.

Instructor shall identify by * those steps considered critical. If step is missed or minimum competency is not met, the evaluated procedure fails and must be repeated.

Performance Criteria	*	Self	Peer	Instructor	Comments
Preparing the Floss					
1. Cuts a piece of floss approximately 18 inches long. Wraps the excess floss around the middle or index fingers of both hands, leaving 2–3 inches of working space exposed.					
2. Stretches the floss tightly between fingers and uses thumb and index finger to guide the floss into place.					
3. Holds the floss tightly between the thumb and forefinger of each hand. The fingers control the floss and should be no farther than 12 inches apart.					
Flossing the Teeth					
1. Passes the floss gently between the patient's teeth, using a sawing motion. Guides the floss to the gumline. Does not force or snap the floss past the contact area.					
2. Curves the floss into a C shape against one tooth. Slides it gently into the space between the gingiva and tooth. Uses both hands to move the floss up and down on one side of the tooth.					
3. Repeats the steps on each side of all the teeth in both arches, including the posterior surface of the last tooth in each quadrant.					

231

Performance Criteria	*	Self	Peer	Instructor	Comments
4. As the floss becomes frayed or soiled, moves a fresh area into the working position.					
Documentation 1. Documents the procedure and results in the patient's chart.					
Additional Comments					

Total number of points possible _____

Total number of points received _____

Grade _____ *Instructor's initials* _____ *Date* _____

COMPETENCY 20-2 APPLYING TOPICAL FLUORIDE GEL OR FOAM (EXPANDED FUNCTION)

Performance Objective

By following a routine procedure that meets stated protocols, the student will be able to apply topical fluoride gel or foam.

Evaluation and Grading Criteria

3   Student competently met the stated criteria without assistance.

2   Student required assistance in order to meet the stated criteria.

1   Student showed uncertainty when performing the stated criteria.

0   Student was not prepared and needs to repeat the step.

N/A   No evaluation of this step.

Instructor shall define grades for each point range earned upon completion of each performance-evaluated task.

Performance Standards

The minimum number of satisfactory performances required prior to final evaluation is _____.

Instructor shall identify by * those steps considered critical. If step is missed or minimum competency is not met, the evaluated procedure fails and must be repeated.

Performance Criteria	*	Self	Peer	Instructor	Comments
Selecting the Tray					
1. Selects a disposable tray that is an appropriate size for the patient's mouth. The tray must be sufficiently long and deep to cover all erupted teeth completely without extending beyond the distal surface of the most posterior tooth.					
Preparing the Teeth					
1. Checks to see whether calculus is present; if not, no preparation is required.					
2. If calculus is present, requests that the dentist or dental hygienist remove it.					
Applying the Topical Fluoride					
1. Seats the patient in an upright position, and explains the procedure.					
2. Instructs the patient not to swallow the fluoride.					
3. Selects the appropriate tray and loads it with a minimal amount of fluoride, following guidelines according to the patient's age.					
4. Dries the teeth using air from the air-water syringe.					
5. Inserts the tray and places cotton rolls between the arches. Asks the patient to bite up and down gently on the cotton rolls.					

233

Performance Criteria	*	Self	Peer	Instructor	Comments
6. Promptly places the saliva ejector and tilts the patient's head forward.					
7. Sets the timer for the appropriate amount of time in accordance with the manufacturer's instructions. Does not leave the patient unattended.					
8. On completion, removes the tray, instructing the patient not to rinse or swallow. Promptly uses the saliva ejector or the high-volume oral evacuator tip to remove excess saliva and solution. Does not allow the patient to close his or her lips tightly around the saliva ejector.					
9. Instructs the patient not to rinse, eat, drink, or brush the teeth for at least 30 minutes.					
Documentation 1. Documents the procedure and outcome in the patient's chart.					
Additional Comments					

Total number of points possible _____

Total number of points received _____

Grade _____ Instructor's initials _____ Date _____

COMPETENCY 20-3 APPLYING FLUORIDE VARNISH (EXPANDED FUNCTION)

Performance objective

By following a routine procedure that meets stated protocols, the student will be able to apply fluoride varnish.

Evaluation and Grading Criteria

3 Student competently met the stated criteria without assistance.

2 Student required assistance in order to meet the stated criteria.

1 Student showed uncertainty when performing the stated criteria.

0 Student was not prepared and needs to repeat the step.

N/A No evaluation of this step.

Instructor shall define grades for each point range earned upon completion of each performance-evaluated task.

Performance Standards

The minimum number of satisfactory performances required prior to final evaluation is _____.

Instructor shall identify by * those steps considered critical. If step is missed or minimum competency is not met, the evaluated procedure fails and must be repeated.

Performance Criteria	*	Self	Peer	Instructor	Comments
1. Obtains informed consent from the patient or parent/legal guardian in the case of a minor patient.					
2. Gathers supplies and single-unit dose for application.					
3. Positions the patient in a supine position.					
4. Wipes the teeth to be varnished with gauze or cotton roll and inserts the saliva ejector.					
5. Using a cotton-tip applicator, brush, or syringe-style applicator, applies 0.3–0.5 mL of varnish (unit dose) to clinical crown of teeth; application time is 1–3 minutes.					
6. Uses dental floss to draw the varnish interproximally.					
7. Allows patient to rinse after the procedure has been completed.					
8. Reminds the patient to avoid eating hard foods, drinking hot or alcoholic beverages, brushing, and flossing for at least 4–6 hours or preferably until the next day after the application. Advises patient to drink through a straw for the first few hours after the application.					

Performance Criteria	*	Self	Peer	Instructor	Comments
Documentation 1. Documents the procedure and results in the patient's chart.					
Additional Comments					

Total number of points possible _____

Total number of points received _____

Grade _____ Instructor's initials _____ Date _____

21 Coronal Polishing and Dental Sealants

TRUE/FALSE

_____ 1. Placement of dental sealants can be a long and uncomfortable procedure for the patient.

_____ 2. The patient, operator, and assistant must use special protective eyewear when the curing light is in use.

_____ 3. Well-placed dental sealants can last more than 10 years with proper care.

_____ 4. Flossing after a coronal polish will help remove any remaining abrasive agent.

_____ 5. Bristle brushes are recommended for use on exposed cementum or dentin.

FILL IN THE BLANK

Select the best term:
  Air-powder polishing
  Calculus
  Clinical crown
  Coronal polish
  Extrinsic
  Fulcrum
  Intrinisic
  Light cured
  Prophylaxis
  Self-cure

6. _____ stains may be removed by scaling or polishing.

7. _____ is a type of sealant material that needs no mixing.

8. A _____ is a finger rest used when performing a coronal polish.

9. A _____ is a procedure in which calculus, debris, stain, and plaque are removed.

10. _____ is a technique that uses a high-pressure stream of water and sodium bicarbonate to remove stain.

11. The _____ is the portion of the tooth that is visible in the mouth.

12. _____ is a type of sealant material that is supplied as a base and catalyst and hardens when mixed together.

13. _____ is a technique used to remove plaque and stains from the coronal surfaces.

14. _____ stains cannot be removed by scaling or polishing.

15. _____ is a hard mineralized deposit on the teeth.

MULTIPLE CHOICE

16. Which of the following is an example of an extrinsic stain?
    a. tobacco stain
    b. dental fluorosis
    c. tetracycline antibiotic stain
    d. all of the above

17. Which of the following is an example of an intrinsic stain?
    a. pulpless teeth
    b. black stain
    c. food and drink
    d. all of the above

18. How do stains occur on teeth?
    a. directly on the surface of the tooth
    b. embedded within the calculus and plaque deposits
    c. incorporated within the tooth structure
    d. all of the above

19. Which of the following is not an indication for requiring dental sealants?
    a. deep pits and fissures
    b. recently erupted tooth
    c. occlusal surface decayed and needs a filling
    d. all of the above

20. Guidelines for sealant placement include:
    a. maintaining a dry tooth surface
    b. preparing the tooth
    c. conditioning the tooth
    d. all of the above

INTERACTIVE DENTAL OFFICE PATIENT CASE EXERCISE

Access the *Interactive Dental Office on Evolve* and click on the patient case file for Todd Ledbetter.
- Review Todd's record.
- Answer the following questions:

1. Which of Todd's teeth are going to have dental sealants?

2. Why did Dr. Roberts not recommend sealants for Todd's anterior teeth?

3. Identify the materials in the sealant setup.

Access the *Interactive Dental Office on Evolve* and click on the patient case file for Christopher Brooks.
- Review Christopher's record.
- Answer the following questions:

1. Which of Christopher's teeth are going to have dental sealants?

2. What type of moisture control is used during sealant placement?

3. Before the sealants are placed, how should the teeth be cleaned?

4. What should be done if Christopher accidentally contaminates the conditioned tooth surface with his saliva?

COMPETENCY 21-1 RUBBER CUP CORONAL POLISHING (EXPANDED FUNCTION)

Performance Objective

By following a routine procedure that meets stated protocols, the student will be able to properly perform rubber cup coronal polishing.

Evaluation and Grading Criteria

3	Student competently met the stated criteria without assistance.
2	Student required assistance in order to meet the stated criteria.
1	Student showed uncertainty when performing the stated criteria.
0	Student was not prepared and needs to repeat the step.
N/A	No evaluation of this step.

Instructor shall define grades for each point range earned upon completion of each performance-evaluated task.

Performance Standards

The minimum number of satisfactory performances required prior to final evaluation is _____.

Instructor shall identify by * those steps considered critical. If step is missed or minimum competency is not met, the evaluated procedure fails and must be repeated.

Performance Criteria	*	Self	Peer	Instructor	Comments
1. Reviews the patient's medical history for contraindications to the coronal polish procedure.					
2. Seats and drapes the patient with a patient napkin. Asks the patient to remove any dental prosthetic appliance that he or she may be wearing. Provides the patient with protective eyewear.					
3. Explains the procedure to the patient and answers any questions.					
4. Inspects oral cavity for lesions, missing teeth, tori, etc.					
5. Applies a disclosing agent to identify areas of plaque.					
Maxillary Right Posterior Quadrant, Buccal Aspect					
1. Sits in the 8 o'clock to 9 o'clock position.					
2. Asks the patient to tilt head up and turn slightly away from the assistant.					
3. Holds the dental mirror in left hand to retract the cheek and for indirect vision of the more posterior teeth.					
4. Establishes a fulcrum on the maxillary right incisors.					
Maxillary Right Posterior Quadrant, Lingual Aspect					
1. Remains seated in the 8 o'clock to 9 o'clock position.					

Performance Criteria	*	Self	Peer	Instructor	Comments
2. Asks the patient to turn head up and toward the assistant.					
3. Holds the dental mirror in left hand for direct vision, providing a view of the distal surfaces.					
4. Establishes a fulcrum on the lower incisors to reach the lingual surfaces.					
Maxillary Anterior Teeth, Facial Aspect					
1. Remains in the 8 o'clock to 9 o'clock position.					
2. Positions the patient's head tipped up slightly and facing straight ahead. Makes necessary adjustments by turning the patient's head either slightly toward or away from the assistant.					
3. Uses direct vision in this area.					
4. Establishes a fulcrum on the incisal edge of the teeth adjacent to the ones being polished.					
Maxillary Anterior Teeth, Lingual Aspect					
1. Remains in the 8 o'clock to 9 o'clock position or moves to the 11 o'clock to 12 o'clock position.					
2. Positions the patient's head so that it is tipped slightly upward.					
3. Uses the mouth mirror for indirect vision and to reflect light on the area.					
4. Establishes a fulcrum on the incisal edge of the teeth adjacent to the ones being polished.					
Maxillary Left Posterior Quadrant, Buccal Aspect					
1. Sits in the 9 o'clock position.					
2. Positions the patient's head tipped upward and turned slightly toward the assistant to improve visibility.					
3. Uses the mirror to retract the cheek and for indirect vision.					
4. Rests fulcrum finger on the buccal occlusal surface of the teeth toward the front of the sextant (or rests fulcrum finger on the lower premolars and reaches the maxillary posterior teeth).					
Maxillary Left Posterior Quadrant, Lingual Aspect					
1. Remains in the 8 o'clock to 9 o'clock position.					
2. Asks the patient to turn head away from the assistant.					

Performance Criteria	*	Self	Peer	Instructor	Comments
3. Uses direct vision in this position. Holds the mirror in left hand for retraction and reflecting light.					
4. Establishes a fulcrum on the buccal surfaces of the maxillary left posterior teeth or on the occlusal surfaces of the mandibular left teeth.					
Maxillary Left Posterior Quadrant, Lingual Aspect 1. Remains in the 8 o'clock to 9 o'clock position.					
2. Asks the patient to turn head away from the assistant.					
3. Uses direct vision in this position. Holds the mirror in left hand for retraction and reflecting light.					
4. Establishes a fulcrum on the buccal surfaces of the maxillary left posterior teeth or on the occlusal surfaces of the mandibular left teeth.					
Mandibular Left Posterior Quadrant, Buccal Aspect 1. Sits in the 8 o'clock to 9 o'clock position.					
2. Asks the patient to turn head slightly toward the assistant.					
3. Uses the mirror to retract the cheek and for indirect vision of distal and buccal surfaces.					
4. Establishes a fulcrum on the incisal surfaces of the mandibular left anterior teeth and reaches back to the posterior teeth.					
Mandibular Left Posterior Quadrant, Lingual Aspect 1. Remains in the 9 o'clock position.					
2. Asks the patient to turn head slightly away from the assistant.					
3. For direct vision, uses the mirror to retract the tongue and reflect more light to the working area.					
4. Establishes a fulcrum on the mandibular anterior teeth and reaches back to the posterior teeth.					
Mandibular Anterior Teeth, Facial Aspect 1. Sits in either the 8 o'clock to 9 o'clock position or in the 11 o'clock to 12 o'clock position.					
2. As necessary, instructs the patient to make adjustments in the head position by turning either toward or away from the assistant or by tilting the head up or down.					
3. Uses left index finger to retract the lower lip. Uses both direct and indirect vision in this area.					

241

Performance Criteria	*	Self	Peer	Instructor	Comments
4. Establishes a fulcrum on the incisal edges of the teeth adjacent to the ones being polished.					
Mandibular Anterior Teeth, Lingual Aspect					
1. Sits in either the 8 o'clock to 9 o'clock position or in the 11 o'clock to 12 o'clock position.					
2. As necessary, instructs the patient to make adjustments in the head position by turning either toward or away from the assistant or by tilting the head up or down.					
3. Uses the mirror for indirect vision, to retract the tongue, and to reflect light onto the teeth.					
4. Establishes a fulcrum on the mandibular canine incisal area.					
Mandibular Right Quadrant, Buccal Aspect					
1. Sits in the 8 o'clock position.					
2. Asks the patient to turn head slightly away from the assistant.					
3. Uses the mirror to retract tissue and reflect light. Also uses mirror to view the distal surfaces in the area.					
4. Establishes a fulcrum on the lower incisors.					
Mandibular Right Quadrant, Lingual Aspect					
1. Remains in the 8 o'clock position.					
2. Asks the patient to turn head slightly toward the assistant.					
3. Retracts the tongue with the mirror.					
4. Establishes a fulcrum on the lower incisors.					
Mandibular Right Quadrant, Lingual Aspect					
1. Sits in the 8 o'clock to 9 o'clock position.					
2. Asks the patient to turn head slightly toward the assistant.					
3. Retracts the tongue with the mirror.					
4. Establishes a fulcrum on the lower incisors.					
Additional Comments					

Total number of points possible _____

Total number of points received _____

Grade _____ *Instructor's initials* _____ *Date* _____

242

Performance Objective

By following a routine procedure that meets stated protocols, the student will be able to apply a light-cured dental sealant according to the manufacturer's instructions and within the scope of the state dental practice act.

Evaluation and Grading Criteria

3	Student competently met the stated criteria without assistance.
2	Student required assistance in order to meet the stated criteria.
1	Student showed uncertainty when performing the stated criteria.
0	Student was not prepared and needs to repeat the step.
N/A	No evaluation of this step.

Instructor shall define grades for each point range earned upon completion of each performance-evaluated task.

Performance Standards

The minimum number of satisfactory performances required prior to final evaluation is _____.

Instructor shall identify by * those steps considered critical. If step is missed or minimum competency is not met, the evaluated procedure fails and must be repeated.

Performance Criteria	*	Self	Peer	Instructor	Comments
1. Teeth are selected by the dentist that have deep pits and fissures and are sufficiently erupted so that a dry field can be maintained.					
2. Checks air-water syringe by blowing a jet of air from the syringe onto a mirror or glove. If small droplets are visible, the syringe is adjusted so that only air is expressed.					
3. Prepares the saliva ejector or high-volume evacuator. Prepares the enamel thoroughly with pumice and water to remove plaque and debris from the occlusal surface. Rinses thoroughly with water.					
4. Isolates and dries the teeth with air syringe and isolates the teeth using either the dental dam or cotton rolls.					
5. Etches the enamel, using the syringe tip or device, to apply a generous amount of etchant to all enamel surfaces to be sealed, extending slightly beyond the anticipated margin of the sealant. Etches for a minimum of 15 seconds but no longer than 60 seconds.					
6. Thoroughly rinses etched teeth with the air-water syringe to remove etchant. Suctions excess water. Does not allow the patient to swallow or rinse.					

243

Performance Criteria	*	Self	Peer	Instructor	Comments
7. Thoroughly dries the etched enamel surfaces using the air-water syringe. The air from the syringe should be dry and free from oil and water. The dry etched surfaces should appear matte, frosty white. If not, repeats steps 5 and 6. Does not allow the etched surface to be contaminated.					
8. Using the syringe tip or brush, slowly applies sealant into the pits and fissures. Does not allow sealant to flow beyond the etched surfaces. Moving the sealant with the syringe tip or brush during or after the placement helps eliminate any bubbles and increases the flow into the pits and fissures. An explorer can also be used. Remembers to check the manufacturer's recommendations for the most effective technique for sealant placement.					
9. To light-cure the sealant, holds the tip of the light as close as possible to the sealant without actually touching the sealant. A 20-second exposure is needed for each surface.					
10. Carefully inspects the sealant for complete coverage and voids. If the surface has not been contaminated, places additional sealant material. If contamination has occurred, re-etches and dries before placing more sealant material. Checks the interproximal areas using dental floss to make certain there is no sealant material in the contact area.					
11. Wipes the sealant with a cotton roll and removes the thin, sticky film on the surface. Checks occlusion using articulating paper and adjusts if required.					
12. Documents the procedure in the patient's chart.					
Additional Comments					

Total number of points possible _____

Total number of points received _____

Grade _____ Instructor's initials _____ Date _____

22 Restorative Dentistry

TRUE/FALSE

_____ 1. Esthetic dentistry is devoted to improving the appearance of a tooth.

_____ 2. The purpose of cavity preparation is to remove decay and a small amount of healthy tooth structure.

_____ 3. Universal matrix bands are made of a soft latex material.

_____ 4. Before assembling the matrix band in its retainer for an amalgam restoration, prepare the band with varnish.

_____ 5. A veneer is a thin layer of tooth-colored material that can be bonded or cemented to the facial surface of a tooth.

_____ 6. A wedge is placed in the embrasure to hold the matrix band firmly against the margin of a preparation and to create a natural contact with its adjacent tooth.

_____ 7. The placement of a retention pin along with bonding material would be indicated to provide strength and retention for the filling material.

_____ 8. Vital bleaching is a technique that involves the whitening of the pulp of the teeth.

_____ 9. The dentist will commonly use hand instruments over rotary instruments to prepare a tooth and place retentive grooves in the preparation.

_____ 10. A clear plastic or Mylar matrix strip is the matrix of choice for Class III and IV anterior restoration.

MATCHING

Match the type of restoration to Black's classification of cavities.

_____ 11. Incisal edge composite   A. Class VI

_____ 12. Occlusal amalgam   B. Class II

_____ 13. Mesial-incisal composite   C. Class I

_____ 14. Distal composite   D. Class III

_____ 15. Mesial-occlusal-distal amalgam   E. Class IV

      F. Class V

_____ 16. Gingival-third composite

SHORT ANSWER

17. Describe a dental condition that would require a restorative dental treatment.

18. Describe a dental condition that would require an esthetic dental treatment.

INTERACTIVE DENTAL OFFICE PATIENT CASE EXERCISE

Access the *Interactive Dental Office* on *Evolve* and click on the patient case file for Miguel Ricardo.

■ Review Mr. Ricardo's record.
■ Complete all exercises on Evolve for Mr. Ricardo's case.
■ Answer the following questions:

1. Which teeth received a matrix in the restoration process?

2. Does Mr. Ricardo have any composite restorations in place at this time?

3. For what restorative procedure should Mr. Ricardo be scheduled?

4. Which tooth will be restored?

5. What type of matrix system will be prepared for the procedure?

COMPETENCY 22-1 ASSEMBLING A MATRIX BAND AND UNIVERSAL RETAINER

Performance Objective

By following a routine procedure that meets stated protocols, the student will be able to assemble a matrix band and universal retainer.

Evaluation and Grading Criteria

3   Student competently met the stated criteria without assistance.

2   Student required assistance in order to meet the stated criteria.

1   Student showed uncertainty when performing the stated criteria.

0   Student was not prepared and needs to repeat the step.

N/A   No evaluation of this step.

Instructor shall define grades for each point range earned upon completion of each performance-evaluated task.

Performance Standards

The minimum number of satisfactory performances required prior to final evaluation is _____.

Instructor shall identify by * those steps considered critical. If step is missed or minimum competency is not met, the evaluated procedure fails and must be repeated.

Performance Criteria	*	Self	Peer	Instructor	Comments
1. Rinses and dries the preparation.					
2. Examines the outline of the cavity preparation using a mirror and explorer.					
3. Determines the size of matrix band to be used for the procedure.					
4. Places the middle of the band on the paper pad and burnishes the area with a burnisher.					
5. Holds the retainer with the diagonal slot facing self and turns the outer knob counterclockwise until the end of the spindle is visible and away from the diagonal slot in the vise.					
6. Turns the inner knob until the vise moves next to the guide slots.					
7. Brings together the ends of the band to identify the occlusal and gingival aspects of the matrix band. The occlusal edge has the larger circumference; the gingival edge has the smaller circumference.					
8. With the diagonal slot of the retainer facing toward self, slides the joined ends of the band, occlusal edge first, into the diagonal slot on the vise.					
9. Guides the band in the correct guide slots.					

247

Performance Criteria	*	Self	Peer	Instructor	Comments
10. Tightens the band and uses the mirror handle to open the band and ready for placement.					
Additional Comments					

Total number of points possible _____

Total number of points received _____

Grade _____ *Instructor's initials* _____ *Date* _____

Performance Objective

By following a routine procedure that meets stated protocols, the student will demonstrate the proper technique for placing and removing a plastic matrix band.

Evaluation and Grading Criteria

3   Student competently met the stated criteria without assistance.

2   Student required assistance in order to meet the stated criteria.

1   Student showed uncertainty when performing the stated criteria.

0   Student was not prepared and needs to repeat the step.

N/A   No evaluation of this step.

Instructor shall define grades for each point range earned upon completion of each performance-evaluated task.

Performance Standards

The minimum number of satisfactory performances required prior to final evaluation is _____.

Instructor shall identify by * those steps considered critical. If step is missed or minimum competency is not met, the evaluated procedure fails and must be repeated.

Performance Criteria	*	Self	Peer	Instructor	Comments
1. Examines the contour of the tooth and preparation site, paying special attention to the outline of the preparation.					
2. Contours the matrix strip.					
3. Slides the matrix interproximal, ensuring that the gingival edge of the matrix extends beyond the preparation.					
4. Using thumb and forefinger, pulls the band over the prepared tooth on the facial and lingual surfaces.					
5. Using cotton pliers, positions the wedge into the gingival embrasure.					
6. Removes the matrix after the preparation was filled and light cured.					
Additional Comments					

Total number of points possible _____

Total number of points received _____

Grade _____ Instructor's initials _____ Date _____

COMPETENCY 22-3 PLACING AND REMOVING A MATRIX BAND AND WEDGE FOR A CLASS II RESTORATION (EXPANDED FUNCTION)

Performance Objective

By following a routine procedure that meets stated protocols, the student will be able to place and remove a matrix band and wedge for a Class II restoration.

Evaluation and Grading Criteria

3   Student competently met the stated criteria without assistance.

2   Student required assistance in order to meet the stated criteria.

1   Student showed uncertainty when performing the stated criteria.

0   Student was not prepared and needs to repeat the step.

N/A   No evaluation of this step.

Instructor shall define grades for each point range earned upon completion of each performance-evaluated task.

Performance Standards

The minimum number of satisfactory performances required prior to final evaluation is _____.

Instructor shall identify by * those steps considered critical. If step is missed or minimum competency is not met, the evaluated procedure fails and must be repeated.

Performance Criteria	*	Self	Peer	Instructor	Comments
Preparing the Band Size					
1. Uses the handle end of the mouth mirror to open the loop of the band.					
2. Adjusts the size (diameter) of the loop to fit over the tooth by turning the inner knob.					
Placing the Matrix Band and Universal Retainer					
1. Positions and seats the loop of the band over the occlusal surface, with the retainer parallel to the buccal surface of the tooth. Ensures the band remains beyond the occlusal edge by approximately 1.0–1.5 mm.					
2. Holds the band securely in place by applying finger pressure over the occlusal surface. Slowly turns the inner knob clockwise to tighten the band around the tooth.					
3. Uses the explorer to examine the adaptation of the band.					
4. Uses a burnisher to contour the band at the contact area, creating a slightly concave area.					
Placing the Wedge					
1. Selects the proper wedge size and shape.					
2. Places the wedge in the pliers so that the flat, wider side of the wedge is toward the gingival embrasure.					
3. Inserts the wedge into the lingual embrasure next to the preparation and the band.					

251

Performance Criteria	*	Self	Peer	Instructor	Comments
4. Checks the proximal contact to ensure that the seal at the gingival margin of the preparation is closed.					
Removing Universal Retainer, Matrix Band, and Wedge					
1. Following the initial carving of the restorative material, loosens the retainer from the band by placing a finger over the occlusal surface and slowly turns the outer knob of the retainer.					
2. Carefully slides the retainer toward the occlusal surface while leaving the band around the tooth.					
3. While grasping both ends of the band, gently lifts the matrix band in an occlusal direction, using a seesaw motion.					
4. Discards the matrix band into the "sharps" container.					
5. Using #110 pliers, grasps the base of the wedge to remove it from the lingual embrasure.					
6. The restoration is now ready for the final carving steps.					
Additional Comments					

Total number of points possible _____

Total number of points received _____

Grade _____ Instructor's initials _____ Date _____

COMPETENCY 22-4 ASSISTING IN A CLASS II AMALGAM RESTORATION

Performance Objective

By following a routine procedure that meets stated protocols, the student will be able to assist in a Class II amalgam restoration.

Evaluation and Grading Criteria

3   Student competently met the stated criteria without assistance.

2   Student required assistance in order to meet the stated criteria.

1   Student showed uncertainty when performing the stated criteria.

0   Student was not prepared and needs to repeat the step.

N/A   No evaluation of this step.

Instructor shall define grades for each point range earned upon completion of each performance-evaluated task.

Performance Standards

The minimum number of satisfactory performances required prior to final evaluation is _____.

Instructor shall identify by ∗ those steps considered critical. If step is missed or minimum competency is not met, the evaluated procedure fails and must be repeated.

Performance Criteria	∗	Self	Peer	Instructor	Comments
Preparing the Tooth 1. Transfers the mouth mirror and explorer to the dentist.					
2. Assists in administration of the local anesthetic agent.					
3. Places and secures moisture control materials (cotton roll, dental dam).					
Preparing the Cavity 1. Transfers the mirror and the high-speed handpiece with cutting bur to the dentist.					
2. During cavity preparation, uses the high-volume evacuator (HVE) and air-water syringe, adjusts the light, and retracts the patient's cheek and tongue as necessary to maintain a clear field for the dentist.					
3. Transfers the explorer, excavators, and hand-cutting instruments as needed throughout the cavity preparation.					
Placing the Base and Cavity Liner (Expanded Function) 1. Rinses and dries the preparation. Mixes and places necessary cavity liners and base.					
Placing the Matrix Band and Wedge (Expanded Function) 1. Assists in placing the preassembled universal (Tofflemire) retainer and matrix.					
2. Assists in placing the wedge or wedges in the proximal box using cotton pliers or #110 pliers.					

253

Performance Criteria	*	Self	Peer	Instructor	Comments
Placing the Bonding Agent (Expanded Function) 1. Assists the dentist in the etching and bonding processes.					
Mixing the Amalgam 1. Activates the capsule, places it in the amalgamator, closes the cover, and sets the timer for the time recommended by the manufacturer.					
2. At the signal from the dentist, starts the amalgamator.					
3. Opens the capsule and removes the pestle with cotton pliers. Drops the amalgam into the amalgam well.					
4. Reassembles and discards the capsule.					
Placing and Condensing the Amalgam 1. Fills the smaller end of the amalgam carrier and transfers the carrier to the dentist.					
2. Assists when necessary as the dentist exchanges the carrier for a condenser and begins condensing the first increments of amalgam with the smaller end of the condenser.					
3. Assists in the process of placing and condensing the amalgam until the cavity is slightly overfilled.					
4. When the cavity preparation is slightly overfilled, exchanges the condenser for the burnisher so that the dentist can burnish the surface and margins of the restoration.					
Initial Carving 1. Assists while the dentist uses the explorer and discoid/cleoid carver to remove the excess amalgam on the occlusal surface, from between the matrix band, and from the marginal ridge of the tooth.					
2. Assists in removing the universal retainer, matrix band, and wedge.					
Final Carving 1. Transfers the amalgam carvers until the carving is complete.					
2. Keeps the tip of the HVE close to the restoration during the carving process.					

Performance Criteria	*	Self	Peer	Instructor	Comments
Occlusal Adjustment 1. Removes moisture control materials (cotton rolls, dental dam).					
2. Prepares articulating paper for the occlusion to be checked, and instructs the patient to close teeth together very gently.					
3. Transfers carver to remove any remaining high spots.					
4. Transfers a moist cotton pellet in cotton pliers and gently rubs the surface of the amalgam.					
Postoperative Instructions 1. Instructs the patient not to chew on the new restoration for a few hours.					
Additional Comments					

Total number of points possible _____

Total number of points received _____

Grade _____ *Instructor's initials* _____ *Date* _____

COMPETENCY 22-5 ASSISTING IN A CLASS III OR IV COMPOSITE RESTORATION

Performance Objective

By following a routine procedure that meets stated protocols, the student will be able to assist in a Class III or IV Restoration.

Evaluation and Grading Criteria

3	Student competently met the stated criteria without assistance.
2	Student required assistance in order to meet the stated criteria.
1	Student showed uncertainty when performing the stated criteria.
0	Student was not prepared and needs to repeat the step.
N/A	No evaluation of this step.

Instructor shall define grades for each point range earned upon completion of each performance-evaluated task.

Performance Standards

The minimum number of satisfactory performances required prior to final evaluation is _____.

Instructor shall identify by * those steps considered critical. If step is missed or minimum competency is not met, the evaluated procedure fails and must be repeated.

Performance Criteria	*	Self	Peer	Instructor	Comments
Preparing the Tooth					
1. Transfers the mouth mirror and explorer to the dentist.					
2. Assists in administration of the local anesthetic.					
3. Assists in selection of the shade of the composite material.					
4. Places and secures moisture control materials (cotton roll, dental dam).					
Preparing the Cavity					
1. Transfers the high-speed handpiece and hand-cutting instruments so the dentist is able to remove decay. Uses the high-volume evacuator (HVE) to maintain a clear operating field.					
2. Rinses and dries the tooth throughout the procedure. If indicated, places a cavity liner.					
Etching, Bonding, and Composite Placement					
1. Assists in the etching according to the manufacturer's instructions. Rinses and dries etched tooth.					
2. Assists in placing the matrix strip. If indicated, a wedge is also placed.					
3. Assists in the application of the primer and bonding resin. Light-cures the material in accordance with the manufacturer's instructions.					
4. Readies the composite syringe material and transfers it along with the composite instrument to be placed in the preparation.					

257

Performance Criteria	*	Self	Peer	Instructor	Comments
5. Light-cures the material from the lingual and facial surfaces.					
Finishing the Restoration 1. Removes the matrix strip and wedge.					
2. Assists with transfers as the dentist used finishing burs or diamonds in the high-speed handpiece to contour the restoration.					
3. If indicated, transfers finishing strips for smoothing the interproximal surface.					
4. Removes the moisture control materials, and readies articulating paper to check the occlusion.					
5. Assists while the dentist uses polishing discs, points, and cups in the low-speed handpiece to polish the restoration.					
Additional Comments					

Total number of points possible _____

Total number of points received _____

Grade _____ *Instructor's initials* _____ *Date* _____

23 Prosthodontics and Digital Technology

TRUE/FALSE

_____ 1. Gingival retraction cord permanently displaces the gingival tissue and widens the sulcus for the permanent restoration.

_____ 2. Provisional coverage is another term used for temporary coverage.

_____ 3. A dental implant is commonly fabricated from titanium.

_____ 4. To ensure an exact color match, many dentists prefer to match the shade of a patient's teeth with the use of fluorescent lighting.

_____ 5. A core buildup can be prepared from either amalgam or a specific core material.

_____ 6. A removable partial denture replaces all of the teeth in an arch.

_____ 7. Anterior teeth are the strongest teeth for abutments of a partial.

_____ 8. Pressure points are areas within the gingival side of a denture that can irritate the patient's tissue.

_____ 9. The use of a gingival retraction cord is not required when taking a final impression for a denture.

_____ 10. An immediate denture is placed immediately after the insertion of an implant.

MATCHING

Match the following types of prostheses to their description:

_____ 11. A fixed prosthesis that covers a portion of the occlusal and proximal surfaces of a tooth

_____ 12. Removable prosthesis that replaces all of the teeth in one arch

_____ 13. Full metal crown with the outer surface covered with a thin layer of tooth-colored material

_____ 14. Prosthesis cemented in place that covers the anatomical portion of an individual tooth

_____ 15. Removable prosthesis that replaces one or more teeth in same arch

_____ 16. A prosthesis cemented in place that replaces one or more adjacent teeth in the same arch

_____ 17. Implant that is surgically placed into the maxilla or mandible that holds one or more prosthetic teeth.

A. Porcelain fused to metal

B. Fixed bridge

C. Endosteal

D. Full denture

E. Full crown

F. Partial denture

G. Onlay

SHORT ANSWER

18. List the indications for a partial denture.

19. Describe osseointegration.

20. Give the three types of an endosteal implant.

INTERACTIVE DENTAL OFFICE PATIENT CASE EXERCISE

Access the *Interactive Dental Office* on *Evolve* and click on the patient case file for Jessica Brooks.
- Review Ms. Brooks's record.
- Complete all exercises on Evolve for Ms. Brooks's case.
- Answer the following questions:

1. Does Ms. Brooks have any existing crown and bridge work?

2. If she was charted to have an amalgam, why did the procedure change to a crown?

3 Why did Ms. Brooks require a core buildup?

4. What type of crown was prescribed for the preparation?

5. Are there any specific oral hygiene procedures that should be given to Ms. Brooks for the care of a crown?

Access the *Interactive Dental Office* on *Evolve* and click on the patient case file for Gregory Brooks.
- Review Mr. Brooks's record.
- Complete all exercises on Evolve for Mr. Brooks's case.
- Answer the following questions:

1. Are there any other types of fixed prosthetics in Mr. Brooks's mouth?

2. Which type of implant did Mr. Brooks decide to have?

3. If Mr. Brooks decided not to proceed with the placement of an implant because of cost, what would be another choice of treatment?

4. What type of home care is recommended for implants?

5. After the implant procedure is completed, what will Mr. Brooks be scheduled for next?

Access the *Interactive Dental Office* on *Evolve* and click on the patient case file for Jose Escobar.
- Review Mr. Escobar's record.
- Complete all exercises on Evolve for Mr. Escobar's case.
- Answer the following questions:

1. How many missing teeth does Mr. Escobar have?

2. What other specialists might have been involved in the development of the treatment plan?

3. Is Mr. Escobar receiving a full or a partial denture?

4. Why were implants not discussed as a possible treatment?

5. Is it possible that Mr. Escobar will need to have his denture relined? Why?

Access the *Interactive Dental Office* on *Evolve* and click on the patient case file for Chester Higgins.
- Review Mr. Higgins's record.
- Complete all exercises on Evolve for Mr. Higgins's case.
- Answer the following questions:

1. Which teeth are involved in the three-unit bridge?

2. What type of provisional was selected to fabricate for this case?

3. Besides an alginate impression, what can be used in fabricating a custom provisional?

4. What common cement would be used for the cementation of the provisional?

5. What type of home care instructions should be provided to the patient for provisional coverage?

COMPETENCY 23-1 PLACING AND REMOVING THE GINGIVAL RETRACTION CORD (EXPANDED FUNCTION)

Performance Objective

By following a routine procedure that meets stated protocols, the student will be able to place and remove a gingival retraction cord.

Evaluation and Grading Criteria

3   Student competently met the stated criteria without assistance.

2   Student required assistance in order to meet the stated criteria.

1   Student showed uncertainty when performing the stated criteria.

0   Student was not prepared and needs to repeat the step.

N/A   No evaluation of this step.

Instructor shall define grades for each point range earned upon completion of each performance-evaluated task.

Performance Standards

The minimum number of satisfactory performances required prior to final evaluation is _____.

Instructor shall identify by * those steps considered critical. If step is missed or minimum competency is not met, the evaluated procedure fails and must be repeated.

Performance Criteria	*	Self	Peer	Instructor	Comments
Preparation					
1. Rinses and gently dries the prepared tooth; isolates the quadrant with cotton rolls.					
2. Cuts a piece of retraction cord 1 to $1^{1/2}$ inches in length, depending on the size and type of tooth being prepared.					
3. Uses cotton pliers to form a loose loop of the cord.					
Placement					
1. Makes a loop in the retraction cord, slips it over the tooth, and positions the loop in the sulcus around the prepared tooth.					
2. Using the cord-packing instrument and working in a clockwise direction, packs the cord gently into the sulcus surrounding the prepared tooth so that the ends are on the facial aspect.					
3. Packs the cord into the sulcus by gently rocking the instrument slightly backward as the instrument is moved forward to the next loose section of retraction cord. Repeats this action until the length of the cord is packed in place.					
4. Overlaps the cord where it meets the first end of the cord. Tucks the ends into the sulcus on the facial aspect.					

263

Performance Criteria	*	Self	Peer	Instructor	Comments
5. Optional: If there is a wider and deeper sulcus, places two retraction cords one on top of the other. Before the impression material is taken, removes the top cord. After the impression is completed, removes the second retraction cord.					
6. Leaves the cord in place for a maximum of 5–7 minutes. Instructs the patient to remain still to keep the area dry.					
Removal 1. Grasps the end of the retraction cord with cotton pliers and removes it in a counterclockwise direction (the reverse of the method used in packing).					
2. Removes the retraction cord just before the impression material is placed.					
3. Gently dries the area and applies fresh cotton rolls.					
Additional Comments					

Total number of points possible _____

Total number of points received _____

Grade _____ *Instructor's initials* _____ *Date* _____

Performance Objective

By following a routine procedure that meets stated protocols, the student will be able to fabricate and cement a custom acrylic provisional crown.

Evaluation and Grading Criteria

3   Student competently met the stated criteria without assistance.

2   Student required assistance in order to meet the stated criteria.

1   Student showed uncertainty when performing the stated criteria.

0   Student was not prepared and needs to repeat the step.

N/A   No evaluation of this step.

Instructor shall define grades for each point range earned upon completion of each performance-evaluated task.

Performance Standards

The minimum number of satisfactory performances required prior to final evaluation is _____.

Instructor shall identify by * those steps considered critical. If step is missed or minimum competency is not met, the evaluated procedure fails and must be repeated.

Performance Criteria	*	Self	Peer	Instructor	Comments
Preliminary Steps					
1. Takes the alginate impression of the arch before the teeth are prepared.					
2. Evaluates the impression, making sure it is free of debris and tears in the area selected for the making of the provisional crown or bridge covering.					
3. Disinfects the impression and keeps it moist until needed.					
4. Isolates the prepared tooth with cotton rolls to maintain moisture control.					
5. Lightly applies separating medium to the prepared tooth to facilitate separating the acrylic from the preparation.					
Mixing and Applying the Acrylic Resin					
1. Places liquid monomer in the mixing container (10 drops of liquid per unit recommended). Quickly dispenses the selected shade of self-curing powder (polymer) into the monomer until the powder is saturated.					
2. Uses a small spatula to blend the powder and liquid into a homogeneous mix.					
3. Sets the mixed material aside for 1–2 minutes until the resin takes on a doughy, less glossy appearance.					
4. Unwraps the alginate impression and gently dries the area corresponding to the teeth that will receive provisional coverage.					

265

Performance Criteria	*	Self	Peer	Instructor	Comments
5. Removes the resin from the mixing container with a small spatula and fills in the prepared tooth space with the material.					
6. Alternatively, if using a syringe material, expresses the acrylic resin from a cartridge directly into the impression.					
Obtaining the Provisional Coverage					
1. Seats the acrylic-loaded impression back into the patient's mouth on the prepared tooth or teeth.					
2. Allows the material to reach an initial set (approximately 3 minutes) and removes the tray from the patient's mouth.					
3. Carefully removes the provisional coverage from the alginate impression and examines the margins and contact areas.					
4. Marks the marginal border and contact points of the provisional coverage with a pencil to provide better visualization.					
5. Using an acrylic bur on the slow speed handpiece, trims the acrylic resin to within 1 mm of the gingival shoulder of the prepared tooth with an acrylic bur or stone.					
6. Seats the provisional coverage and checks the occlusion, accuracy, and completeness of the provisional coverage on the prepared tooth.					
7. Removes the provisional coverage and polishes with a sterile white rag wheel and pumice on the laboratory lathe.					
8. Temporarily cements the provisional coverage with zinc oxide–eugenol (TempBond™) or intermediate restorative material.					
9. Checks the occlusion with articulating paper. If any reductions are required, assists the dentist using an acrylic-trimming bur.					
Additional Comments					

Total number of points possible _____

Total number of points received _____

Grade _____ *Instructor's initials* _____ *Date* _____

Performance Objective

By following a routine procedure that meets stated protocols, the student will be able to assist in a crown and bridge restoration.

Evaluation and Grading Criteria

3   Student competently met the stated criteria without assistance.

2   Student required assistance in order to meet the stated criteria.

1   Student showed uncertainty when performing the stated criteria.

0   Student was not prepared and needs to repeat the step.

N/A   No evaluation of this step.

Instructor shall define grades for each point range earned upon completion of each performance-evaluated task.

Performance Standards

The minimum number of satisfactory performances required prior to final evaluation is _____.

Instructor shall identify by * those steps considered critical. If step is missed or minimum competency is not met, the evaluated procedure fails and must be repeated.

Performance Criteria	*	Self	Peer	Instructor	Comments
Preliminary Steps					
1. Assists in the administration of the local anesthetic agent.					
2. If an alginate impression is required to fabricate the provisional coverage, obtains the impression at this time. In addition, obtains a bite registration.					
3. If a silicone two-step impression method is used, obtains the first impression at this time.					
4. If this procedure involves the fabrication of a tooth-colored restoration, selects the shade at this time.					
Tooth Preparation					
1. Throughout the preparation, maintains a clear field by using the high-volume evacuator to retract the lips and tongue and remove water and debris.					
2. Assists in bur changes as necessary while the dentist reduces tooth bulk and completes the preparation using different-shaped burs.					
Final Impression					
1. Assists in the placement of the gingival retraction cord.					
2. Assists in readying the final impression material.					
3. Before transferring the light-bodied material, transfers cotton pliers for the dentist to remove the gingival retraction cord.					

Performance Criteria	*	Self	Peer	Instructor	Comments
4. While the dentist is applying the light-bodied material, readies the tray with heavy-bodied material.					
5. Applies air around the material before the dentist seats the impression tray.					
6. Retrieves the light-bodied syringe from the dentist and transfers the tray, ensuring that the dentist can grasp the handle and insert the tray properly.					
7. After the recommended time for the material to set, assists the dentist in removing the tray.					
8. The occlusal registration is obtained.					
Preparing and Cementing the Provisional 1. Provisional coverage is fabricated using the preliminary impression.					
2. Seats the provisional and adjusts prior to temporary cementing.					
3. Has the dentist evaluate the provisional prior to cementation.					
4. Prepares the temporary cement, fills the crown, and places it over the preparation, instructing the patient to bite down on a cotton roll till material sets.					
5. Dismisses the patient and instructs him or her to schedule a cementation appointment.					
6. Provides the dentist with a laboratory prescription and prepares the case to be delivered to the laboratory.					
Additional Comments					

Total number of points possible _____

Total number of points received _____

Grade _____ *Instructor's initials* _____ *Date* _____

COMPETENCY 23-4 ASSISTING IN THE DELIVERY AND CEMENTATION OF A CAST RESTORATION

Performance Objective

By following a routine procedure that meets stated protocols, the student will be able to assist in the delivery and cementation of a cast restoration.

Evaluation and Grading Criteria

3	Student competently met the stated criteria without assistance.
2	Student required assistance in order to meet the stated criteria.
1	Student showed uncertainty when performing the stated criteria.
0	Student was not prepared and needs to repeat the step.
N/A	No evaluation of this step.

Instructor shall define grades for each point range earned upon completion of each performance-evaluated task.

Performance Standards

The minimum number of satisfactory performances required prior to final evaluation is _____.

Instructor shall identify by * those steps considered critical. If step is missed or minimum competency is not met, the evaluated procedure fails and must be repeated.

Performance Criteria	*	Self	Peer	Instructor	Comments
1. Assists the dentist in removing the temporary coverage.					
2. Rinses and dries the preparation and places cotton rolls.					
3. Transfers the cast restoration to the dentist for a try in. Transfers mirror and explorer.					
4. Readies the high-speed handpiece with finishing burs and articulating paper for final evaluation.					
5. Mixes the permanent cement at the signal from dentist, according to the manufacturer's instructions.					
6. Lines the cement on the internal surface of the casting.					
7. Transfers the prepared crown in the palm of the hand, making it easy for the dentist to grasp.					
8. Has a cotton roll ready to transfer after the dentist for the patient to bite down.					
9. Instructs the patient to continue biting down until the cement reaches the initial set, approximately 8–10 minutes.					
10. After cement sets, removes the cotton roll and rinses and dries area.					
11. Uses an explorer to remove the excess cement carefully from the crown.					
12. Applies a fulcrum during cement removal.					

269

Performance Criteria	*	Self	Peer	Instructor	Comments
13. Places the tip of the explorer at the gingival edge of the cement and uses overlapping horizontal strokes to remove the bulk of the cement.					
14. Applies slight lateral pressure (toward the tooth surface) to remove the remaining cement.					
15. Uses dental floss with a tied knot between the teeth to remove excess cement from the interproximal areas.					
16. After the excess cement has been removed, the dentist examines the area.					
Additional Comments					

Total number of points possible _____

Total number of points received _____

Grade _____ *Instructor's initials* _____ *Date* _____

Performance Objective

By following a routine procedure that meets stated protocols, the student will be able to assist in the delivery of a partial denture.

Evaluation and Grading Criteria

3	Student competently met the stated criteria without assistance.
2	Student required assistance in order to meet the stated criteria.
1	Student showed uncertainty when performing the stated criteria.
0	Student was not prepared and needs to repeat the step.
N/A	No evaluation of this step.

Instructor shall define grades for each point range earned upon completion of each performance-evaluated task.

Performance Standards

The minimum number of satisfactory performances required prior to final evaluation is _____.

Instructor shall identify by * those steps considered critical. If step is missed or minimum competency is not met, the evaluated procedure fails and must be repeated.

Performance Criteria	*	Self	Peer	Instructor	Comments
1. Seats the patient.					
2. Assists the dentist in placing the partial denture in the patient's mouth, and instructs the patient to close his or her teeth together.					
3. Assists in checking occlusion by placing articulating paper on the occlusal surface of the mandibular teeth and asking the patient to simulate chewing motions. Readies the handpiece if the occlusion requires adjustment.					
4. Readies pressure-indicator paste to be applied on the tissue surface of the prosthesis. This detects pressure points (high spots) that could cause discomfort to the patient.					
5. The prosthesis is placed in the patient's mouth. Any adjustments are made by the dentist.					
6. Readies the pliers for any adjustments to the tension on the retainers.					
7. Polishes the partial denture on the laboratory lathe, using the appropriate pastes and sterile buffing wheels.					
8. Scrubs the partial denture with soap, water, and a brush; disinfects and rinses it; and returns it to the treatment room for delivery to the patient.					

Performance Criteria	*	Self	Peer	Instructor	Comments
9. Instructs the patient in the placement, removal, and care of the partial denture.					
Additional Comments					

Total number of points possible _____

Total number of points received _____

Grade _____ Instructor's initials _____ Date _____

Performance Objective

By following a routine procedure that meets stated protocols, the student will be able to assist in the delivery of a full denture.

Evaluation and Grading Criteria

3	Student competently met the stated criteria without assistance.
2	Student required assistance in order to meet the stated criteria.
1	Student showed uncertainty when performing the stated criteria.
0	Student was not prepared and needs to repeat the step.
N/A	No evaluation of this step.

Instructor shall define grades for each point range earned upon completion of each performance-evaluated task.

Performance Standards

The minimum number of satisfactory performances required prior to final evaluation is _____.

Instructor shall identify by * those steps considered critical. If step is missed or minimum competency is not met, the evaluated procedure fails and must be repeated.

Performance Criteria	*	Self	Peer	Instructor	Comments
1. Seats the patient.					
2. Assists in the seating of the denture into the patient's mouth. The shade and shape of the artificial teeth are checked for natural appearance.					
3. Instructs the patient to perform facial expressions and the actions of swallowing, chewing, and speaking, using "s" and "th" sounds.					
4. Prepares articulating paper and holder to check occlusion.					
5. Readies the straight handpiece with a finishing stone for adjustments.					
6. Tries the denture in the mouth again until the cusps appear to be in occlusion with the opposing arch.					
7. Schedules appointment with the patient for postdelivery.					
8. Provides the patient with written and oral instructions on wearing and caring for the denture.					
Additional Comments					

Total number of points possible _____

Total number of points received _____

Grade _____ *Instructor's initials* _____ *Date* _____

273

COMPETENCY 23-7 ASSISTING IN AN ENDOSTEAL IMPLANT SURGERY

Performance Objective

By following a routine procedure that meets stated protocols, the student will demonstrate the proper techniques to be used when assisting during the stages of implant surgery.

Evaluation and Grading Criteria

3   Student competently met the stated criteria without assistance.

2   Student required assistance in order to meet the stated criteria.

1   Student showed uncertainty when performing the stated criteria.

0   Student was not prepared and needs to repeat the step.

N/A   No evaluation of this step.

Instructor shall define grades for each point range earned on completion of each performance-evaluated task.

Performance Standards

The minimum number of satisfactory performances required before final evaluation is _____.

Instructor shall identify by * those steps considered critical. If step is missed or minimum competency is not met, the evaluated procedure fails and must be repeated.

Performance Criteria	*	Self	Peer	Instructor	Comment
1. Gathers the appropriate setup.					
2. Places personal protective equipment according to procedure.					
3. Assists in stage I surgery: implant placement.					
4. Maintains patient comfort and follows appropriate infection control measures throughout the procedure.					
5. Assists in stage II surgery: implant exposure.					
6. Maintains patient comfort and follows appropriate infection control measures throughout the procedure.					
7. Documents procedure in patient record.					
Additional Comments					

Total number of points possible _____

Total number of points received _____

Grade _____ *Instructor's initials* _____ *Date* _____

24 Periodontics

TRUE/FALSE

_____ 1. Kirkland knives are included in the peri-odontal surgical tray setup

_____ 2. Ultrasonic scalers are contraindicated because they increase operator hand fatigue.

_____ 3. Fluoride mouth rinses have been shown to reduce bleeding by delaying bacterial growth in periodontal pockets.

_____ 4. The scaling of teeth follows the root planing procedure in order to remove remaining calculus.

_____ 5. A gingivoplasty involves the surgical reshaping and contouring of gingival tissues.

FILL IN THE BLANK

Select the best term:
Explorer
Gingivitis
Gracey
Orban
Periodontitis
Periodontal disease
Periodontal pockets
Pocket marker
Scaler
Universal

6. _____ is an infection that begins in the gingivae and progresses into the alveolar bone.

7. _____ is inflammation of the gingiva.

8. _____ occurs when the sulcus becomes deeper than normal.

9. A _____ is an instrument that is used to remove supragingival calculus.

10. _____ is the leading cause of tooth loss in adults.

11. A _____ curette is an instrument that is area specific and has one cutting edge.

12. A _____ is used to make bleeding points before a gingivectomy.

13. A _____ curette is an instrument with two cutting edges.

14. An _____ is an instrument that provides tactile information to the operator concerning the surface of the root.

15. An _____ knife is used to remove tissue from the interdental areas.

MULTIPLE CHOICE

16. Which of the following are indications for periodontal surgery?
    a. reduce or eliminate pockets
    b. treat defects in the bone
    c. create new tissue attachment
    d. all of the above

17. _____ is a periodontal surgical procedure to remove bone?
    a. gingival graft
    b. laterally sliding flap
    c. osteoplasty
    d. ostectomy

18. Periodontal dressing is prescribed to:
    a. hold gingival flaps in place during healing
    b. protect a surgical site
    c. support mobile teeth during the healing process
    d. all of the above

19. The type of dental material(s) selected for periodontal dressings include:
    a. zinc oxide and eugenol
    b. zinc phosphate
    c. non-eugenol
    d. a and c

20. A postoperative appointment following periodontal surgery should be scheduled approximately:
    a. 24 hours
    b. 48 hours
    c. 1 week
    d. 1 month

Access the Interactive Dental Office on Evolve and click on the patient case for Louisa Van Doren.
- Review Mrs. Van Doren's record.
- Mount her radiographs.
- Answer the following questions:

1. Does Mrs. Van Doren's health history contain any information regarding a condition that could lead to periodontal complications?

2. While viewing Mrs. Van Doren's radiographs, what did you notice about the level of bone?

Access the Interactive Dental Office on Evolve and click on the patient case file for Mrs. Louisa Van Doren.
- Review Mrs. Van Doren's record.
- Complete all exercises for Mrs. Van Doren's case.
- Answer the following questions:

1. Are there contraindications to the use of an ultrasonic scaler on Mrs. Van Doren?

2. A gingivectomy is scheduled for which area in Mrs. Van Doren's mouth?

3. Will Dr. Bowman need to place a periodontal dressing?

Access the Interactive Dental Office on Evolve and click on the patient case file for Mrs. Janet Folkner.
- Review Mrs. Folkner's record.
- Complete all exercises for Mrs. Folkner's case.
- Answer the following questions:

1. Are there any special precautions that should be taken before an ultrasonic scaler is used on Mrs. Folkner?

2. What do you notice regarding the level of bone on Mrs. Folkner's radiographs?

3. What type of instruments would be used to remove the subgingival calculus?

Performance Objective

By following a routine procedure that meets stated protocols, the student will be able to assist competently with a dental prophylaxis procedure.

Evaluation and Grading Criteria

3	Student competently met the stated criteria without assistance.
2	Student required assistance in order to meet the stated criteria.
1	Student showed uncertainty when performing the stated criteria.
0	Student was not prepared and needs to repeat the step.
N/A	No evaluation of this step.

Instructor shall define grades for each point range earned upon completion of each performance-evaluated task.

Performance Standards

The minimum number of satisfactory performances required prior to final evaluation is _____.

Instructor shall identify by * those steps considered critical. If step is missed or minimum competency is not met, the evaluated procedure fails and must be repeated.

Performance Criteria	*	Self	Peer	Instructor	Comments
1. Assists the operator using the air/water syringe to locate interproximal and subgingival calculus.					
2. Uses the high-volume evacuator as necessary and retracts the lips, tongue, and cheeks to improve visibility and access as the operator uses scalers and curettes to remove all calculus and plaque.					
3. Readies a sterile cotton gauze for the operator to remove any remaining calculus.					
4. Assists the operator while coronal polishing the teeth using polishing paste, a rubber cup, and bristle brushes.					
5. Assists the operator to remove any remaining interproximal debris with dental floss or tape.					
6. Provides oral hygiene instructions appropriate to the individual needs of the patient.					
Additional Comments					

Total number of points possible _____

Total number of points received _____

Grade _____ *Instructor's initials* _____ *Date* _____

COMPETENCY 24-2 ASSISTING WITH GINGIVECTOMY AND GINGIVOPLASTY

Performance objective

By following a routine procedure that meets stated protocols, the student will be able to assist the dentist competently in performing gingivectomy and gingivoplasty periodontal procedures.

Evaluation and Grading Criteria

3   Student competently met the stated criteria without assistance.

2   Student required assistance in order to meet the stated criteria.

1   Student showed uncertainty when performing the stated criteria.

0   Student was not prepared and needs to repeat the step.

N/A   No evaluation of this step.

Instructor shall define grades for each point range earned upon completion of each performance-evaluated task.

Performance Standards

The minimum number of satisfactory performances required prior to final evaluation is _____.

Instructor shall identify by * those steps considered critical. If step is missed or minimum competency is not met, the evaluated procedure fails and must be repeated.

Performance Criteria	*	Self	Peer	Instructor	Comments
Role of the Dental Assistant					
1. Sets out the patient's health history, radiographs, and periodontal chart.					
2. Assists in the administration of local anesthetic.					
3. Anticipates the dentist's needs and is prepared to transfer and retrieve surgical instruments when needed.					
4. Has gauze ready to remove tissue from the instruments, as necessary.					
5. Provides oral evacuation and retraction.					
6. Irrigates with sterile saline.					
7. If sutures are used, prepares the suture needle and suture material, and positions them in a hemostat or needle holder. Transfers them to the dentist when requested.					
8. Places, or assists with placement of, the periodontal dressing.					
9. Wipes any blood or debris from the patient's face. Provides postoperative instructions to the patient.					
Role of the Dentist					
1. Administers the local anesthetic.					
2. Marking the pockets on both the facial and the lingual gingivae by using the periodontal pocket marker.					

Performance Criteria	*	Self	Peer	Instructor	Comments
3. Uses a scalpel or periodontal knife to incise the gingiva at a 45-degree angle, following along the bleeding points. The incision is beveled to create a normally contoured, free gingival margin.					
4. Removes the gingival tissue along the incision line using surgical knives.					
5. Tapers the gingival margins and creates a scalloped marginal outline.					
6. Shapes the interdental papillae using interdental knives.					
7. Performs scaling and root planing of the root surfaces.					
8. Places sutures if needed.					
9. Irrigates the surgical site and then covers it with a periodontal dressing.					
Additional Comments					

Total number of points possible _____

Total number of points received _____

Grade _____ *Instructor's initials* _____ *Date* _____

COMPETENCY 24-3 PREPARING AND PLACING NONEUGENOL PERIODONTAL DRESSING

Performance Objective

By following a routine procedure that meets stated protocols, the student will be able to prepare and assist the dentist in placing a noneugenol periodontal dressing.

Evaluation and Grading Criteria

3   Student competently met the stated criteria without assistance.

2   Student required assistance in order to meet the stated criteria.

1   Student showed uncertainty when performing the stated criteria.

0   Student was not prepared and needs to repeat the step.

N/A   No evaluation of this step.

Instructor shall define grades for each point range earned upon completion of each performance-evaluated task.

Performance Standards

The minimum number of satisfactory performances required prior to final evaluation is _____.

Instructor shall identify by * those steps considered critical. If step is missed or minimum competency is not met, the evaluated procedure fails and must be repeated.

Performance Criteria	*	Self	Peer	Instructor	Comments
Mixing the Material					
1. Extrudes equal lengths of the two pastes on the paper pad.					
2. Mixes the pastes with a wooden tongue depressor until a uniform color is obtained (2–3 minutes).					
3. When the paste loses its tackiness, places it in the paper cup filled with room-temperature water.					
4. Lubricates gloved fingers with saline solution.					
5. Rolls the paste into strips approximately the length of the surgical site.					
Placing the Dressing					
1. Presses small, triangle-shaped pieces of dressing into the interproximal spaces.					
2. Adapts one end of the strip around the distal surface of the last tooth in the surgical site.					
3. Brings the remainder of the strip forward along the facial surface and gently presses the strip along the incised gingival margin.					
4. Gently presses the strip into the interproximal areas.					
5. Applies the second strip in the same manner from the lingual side.					
6. Joins the facial and lingual strips at the distal surface of the last tooth at both ends of the surgical site.					

283

Performance Criteria	*	Self	Peer	Instructor	Comments
7. Applies gentle pressure on the facial and lingual surfaces.					
8. Checks the dressing for overextension and interference with occlusion.					
9. Removes any excess dressing and adjusts the new margins to remove any roughness.					
Additional Comments					

Total number of points possible _____

Total number of points received _____

Grade _____ *Instructor's initials* _____ *Date* _____

COMPETENCY 24-4 REMOVING A PERIODONTAL DRESSING

Performance Objective

By following a routine procedure that meets stated protocols, the student will be able to remove a periodontal dressing.

Evaluation and Grading Criteria

3   Student competently met the stated criteria without assistance.

2   Student required assistance in order to meet the stated criteria.

1   Student showed uncertainty when performing the stated criteria.

0   Student was not prepared and needs to repeat the step.

N/A   No evaluation of this step.

Instructor shall define grades for each point range earned upon completion of each performance-evaluated task.

Performance Standards

The minimum number of satisfactory performances required prior to final evaluation is _____.

Instructor shall identify by * those steps considered critical. If step is missed or minimum competency is not met, the evaluated procedure fails and must be repeated.

Performance Criteria	*	Self	Peer	Instructor	Comments
1. Gently inserts the spoon excavator under the margin.					
2. Uses lateral pressure to pry the dressing gently away from the tissue.					
3. If sutures are embedded in the dressing material, cuts the suture material free. Removes the sutures gently from the tissue.					
4. Gently uses dental floss to remove all fragments of dressing material from the interproximal surfaces.					
5. Irrigates the entire area gently with warm saline solution to remove superficial debris.					
6. Uses the high-volume evacuator tip or saliva ejector to remove the fluid from the patient's mouth.					
Additional Comments					

Total number of points possible _____

Total number of points received _____

Grade _____ Instructor's initials _____ Date _____

25 Endodontics

TRUE/FALSE

_____ 1. Endodontics is a specialty that is dedicated to treating the pulp of the tooth.

_____ 2. A control tooth should be used for each type of pulp testing procedure.

_____ 3. If decay is close to the pulp but has not penetrated it, the condition is termed irreversible pulpitis.

_____ 4. Necrosis is also referred to as "nonvital."

_____ 5. Amalgam is the preferred material to obturate the pulpal canal.

_____ 6. Formocresol is a type of technique used for the pulpotomy of permanent teeth.

_____ 7. A direct pulp cap is indicated when the pulp has been slightly exposed.

_____ 8. A pulpectomy is also referred to as "root canal therapy."

_____ 9. If a tooth is nonvital, the patient may not require the area to be anesthetized for the procedure.

_____ 10. The standard of care established by the ADA for endodontic treatment requires the use of a dental dam for infection control.

MATCHING

Match the following vitality tests with their descriptions:

_____ 11. Tapping on the tooth

_____ 12. Decreased temperature placed on the tooth

_____ 13. Small current to the tooth

_____ 14. Firm pressure to the tooth

_____ 15. Increased temperature to the tooth

A. Electric pulp test

B. Palpation test

C. Heat test

D. Percussion test

E. Cold test

Match the following instruments with their uses:

_____ 16. Hand instrument used to enter and locate canal openings

_____ 17. Paddle-shaped instrument for placement of a temporary restoration

_____ 18. Hand instrument used to condense and adapt gutta-percha points to the canal

_____ 19. Tiny fishhook barbs used to remove the bulk of the pulp tissue

_____ 20. Hand instrument used to obturate the canal by packing the gutta-percha points in a lateral direction

A. Endodontic spreader

B. Broach

C. Endodontic explorer

D. Glick #1

E. Endodontic plugger

SHORT ANSWER

21. The subjective portion of the endodontic examination includes evaluation of symptoms or problems described by the patient. List three specific questions to ask a patient.

22. Radiographic images are exposed a minimum of four times at key points throughout an endodontic procedure. Name and describe each of the four radiographic exposures.

Access the *Interactive Dental Office* on *Evolve* and click on the patient case file for Crystal Malone.
■ Review Ms. Malone's file.
■ Complete all exercises on Evolve for Ms. Malone's case.
■ Answer the following questions:

1. Define the number of teeth that have the following classifications restored: class I, II, III, IV.

2. Does Ms. Malone have any composite restorations in place at this time?

3. For what restorative procedure should Ms. Malone be scheduled?

4. Ms. Malone discovers that her insurance does not cover whitening, and she cannot afford to have the procedure completed at this time. What would be an alternative that the dental team could educate Ms. Malone about?

5. Ms. Malone had tooth #19 restored with a root canal and porcelain-fused-to-metal crown. What dental specialists might have been involved in this restoration process?

Access the *Interactive Dental Office* on *Evolve* and click on the patient case file for Antonio DeAngelis.
■ Review Mr. DeAngelis's record.
■ Complete all exercises on Evolve for Mr. DeAngelis's case.
■ Answer the following questions:

1. Does Mr. DeAngelis have any existing root canals charted?

2. What tooth was used as a control tooth for electric pulp testing?

3. How would tooth #10 be charted after completion of the root canal?

4. What specialist will Mr. DeAngelis be referred to for the porcelain-fused-to-metal crown?

5. Now that the existing work is completed, should Mr. DeAngelis be rescheduled for anything?

Performance Objective

By following a routine procedure that meets stated protocols, the student will be able to assist in an electric pulp vitality test.

Evaluation and Grading Criteria

3   Student competently met the stated criteria without assistance.

2   Student required assistance in order to meet the stated criteria.

1   Student showed uncertainty when performing the stated criteria.

0   Student was not prepared and needs to repeat the step.

N/A   No evaluation of this step.

Instructor shall define grades for each point range earned upon completion of each performance-evaluated task.

Performance Standards

The minimum number of satisfactory performances required prior to final evaluation is _____.

Instructor shall identify by ∗ those steps considered critical. If step is missed or minimum competency is not met, the evaluated procedure fails and must be repeated.

Performance Criteria	∗	Self	Peer	Instructor	Comments
1. Gathers the appropriate setup.					
2. Places personal protective equipment according to procedure.					
3. Describes the procedure to the patient and explains he or she may feel a tingling or a warm sensation.					
4. Identifies the teeth to be tested (suspect tooth and control tooth) and then isolates the teeth and thoroughly dries the area.					
5. Sets the dial (current level) at zero.					
6. Places a thin layer of toothpaste on the tip of the pulp tester electrode.					
7. Tests the control tooth first.					
8. Places the tip of the electrode on the facial surface of the tooth at the cervical third.					
9. Gradually increases the level of the current until the patient feels a sensation. Documents on the patient's record the level at which the response occurs.					
10. Repeats the procedure on the suspect tooth and records the reading.					
Additional Comments					

Total number of points possible _____

Total number of points received _____

Grade _____ Instructor's initials _____ Date _____

Performance Objective

By following a routine procedure that meets stated protocols, the student will be able to assist in root canal therapy.

Evaluation and Grading Criteria

3   Student competently met the stated criteria without assistance.

2   Student required assistance in order to meet the stated criteria.

1   Student showed uncertainty when performing the stated criteria.

0   Student was not prepared and needs to repeat the step.

N/A   No evaluation of this step.

Instructor shall define grades for each point range earned upon completion of each performance-evaluated task.

Performance Standards

The minimum number of satisfactory performances required prior to final evaluation is _____.

Instructor shall identify by * those steps considered critical. If step is missed or minimum competency is not met, the evaluated procedure fails and must be repeated.

Performance Criteria	*	Self	Peer	Instructor	Comments
1. Gathers the appropriate setup.					
2. Place personal protective equipment according to procedure.					
Preparing the Field of Operation					
1. Assists in administration of the local anesthetic agent (if applicable).					
2. Assists with preparation and placement of the dental dam (exposes only the tooth being treated).					
3. Swabs the antiseptic solution over the exposed tooth, the clamp, and the surrounding dental dam.					
Removing the Pulp					
1. Places the HVE tip as the dentist enters the coronal portion of the tooth with a carbide bur, removing decay and infected tooth structure.					
2. Once the canals are located with the endodontic explorer, the pulp tissue is removed with intracanal instruments.					
3. Irrigates the canals gently with the sodium hypochlorite solution. Excess solution is removed with the high-volume evacuator tip.					
4. The dentist uses a small endodontic file to rub the irrigation solution against the walls of the canal and pulp chamber.					
Cleaning and Shaping the Canal					
1. The dentist measures the canals and instructs at what length each file should have the rubber stops placed.					

291

Performance Criteria	*	Self	Peer	Instructor	Comments
2. Transfers each size of file from smaller to larger to the dentist to clean and shape the canals.					
3. Irrigates the canals thoroughly at frequent intervals during this shaping and cleaning process.					
4. Transfers paper points for insertion into the canals until the points come out dry.					
Preparing to Fill the Canal 1. Selects the appropriate-sized gutta-percha point and cuts it to the predetermined length. This is called the trial point.					
2. Takes a periapical radiograph exposure of the tooth with the trial point in the canal. This is the working-length radiograph.					
3. If the exposure does not show the tip of the trial point within 1 mm of the apex of the root, the point is repositioned and another exposure is taken.					
4. At the signal from the dentist, prepares a thin mix of sealer on a sterile glass slab.					
Filling the Canal 1. The master cone is removed from the canal, coated with sealer, and reinserted by the dentist.					
2. The dentist inserts the finger spreader into the canal within 1 mm of the working length. The spreader is rotated counterclockwise to spread the sealer around the canal and create space for the other cones.					
3. Continues transferring gutta-percha points to fill the canal.					
4. Transfers the Glick #1, heated at the working end, to remove the excess ends of the gutta-percha points.					
5. Transfers the plugger for the dentist to compact vertically.					
6. This continues until the canal is completely filled.					
7. The dentist places a temporary restoration.					
8. Exposes a post-treatment radiograph.					
9. The dentist checks the occlusion and adjusts as needed.					

Performance Criteria	*	Self	Peer	Instructor	Comments
Posttreatment Instructions and Follow-up					
1. Instructs the patient to call immediately if there are indications of swelling or pain.					
2. Instructs the patient to return to his or her regular dentist to have a final restoration placed.					
3. Reschedules the patient for follow-up at intervals ranging from 3 to 6 months.					
Additional Comments					

Total number of points possible _____

Total number of points received _____

Grade _____ *Instructor's initials* _____ *Date* _____

26 Oral and Maxillofacial Surgery

TRUE/FALSE

_____ 1. Because of requiring a sterile environment, surgical procedures must take place in the operating room within a hospital setting.

_____ 2. Surgical instruments are classified as critical instruments and are disinfected after each use.

_____ 3. "Luxate" means to rock back and forth to dislocate.

_____ 4. Contact with anything that is not sterile will break the chain of asepsis and contaminate the surgical area.

_____ 5. A forceps extraction is a type of procedure executed on a tooth that is fully impacted.

_____ 6. Alveoloplasty is a procedure of surgically contouring and smoothing the remaining bone in the extraction area to provide a properly contoured ridge.

_____ 7. As a rule, if a scalpel has been used to incise tissue, then sutures are placed for proper healing.

_____ 8. Failure of a blood clot from an extraction can result in alveolitis.

_____ 9. After a surgical procedure, home-care instructions should be provided over the telephone once the patient has arrived home.

_____ 10. Nonabsorbable suture materials include plain catgut, chromic catgut, and polydioxanone.

MATCHING

Match each surgical instrument to its use.

_____ 11. Trims alveolar bone

_____ 12. Removes root tips or fragments of teeth

_____ 13. Separates periosteum from bone

_____ 14. Grasps and holds items

_____ 15. Surgical knife

A. Periosteal elevator
B. Scalpel
C. Rongeur
D. Root tip picks
E. Hemostat

Match the surgical situation with its dental term.

_____ 16. Dry socket

_____ 17. Covered by tissue or bone

_____ 18. Aseptic principle

_____ 19. Examination of questionable area

_____ 20. Recontouring tissue and bone

A. Alveolitis
B. Biopsy
C. Alveoloplasty
D. Impaction
E. Sterile technique

SHORT ANSWER

21. What type of instructions are provided to a patient to controlling bleeding after an extraction?

22. What type of instructions are provided to a patient to controlling swelling?

23. Give the probable causes of alveolitis.

Access the *Interactive Dental Office on Evolve*, and click on the patient case file for Mr. Lee Wong.
- Review Mr. Wong's record.
- Answer the following questions:

1. What does the charting indicate for tooth #30?

2. Could any additional methods of pain control be used to calm Mr. Wong?

3. What type of PPE was worn during the procedure?

4. Were sutures placed after the extraction?

5. How is the medicated dressing placed in the tooth socket for the treatment of alveolitis?

Performance Objective

By following a routine procedure that meets stated protocols, the student will be able to perform a surgical scrub.

Evaluation and Grading Criteria

3   Student competently met the stated criteria without assistance.

2   Student required assistance in order to meet the stated criteria.

1   Student showed uncertainty when performing the stated criteria.

0   Student was not prepared and needs to repeat the step.

N/A   No evaluation of this step.

Instructor shall define grades for each point range earned upon completion of each performance-evaluated task.

Performance Standards

The minimum number of satisfactory performances required prior to final evaluation is _____.

Instructor shall identify by * those steps considered critical. If step is missed or minimum competency is not met, the evaluated procedure fails and must be repeated.

Performance Criteria	*	Self	Peer	Instructor	Comments
1. Covers hair and places protective eyewear and mask before performing a surgical scrub.					
2. Removes all jewelry.					
3. With water running, uses the orange stick to clean under nails. Discards the stick and rinses hands without touching the faucet or inside of the sink.					
4. Wets hands and forearms up to the elbows with warm water and then dispenses about 5 mL of antimicrobial soap into cupped hands.					
5. Uses the surgical scrub brush to scrub hands and forearms for 7 minutes.					
6. Rinses thoroughly with warm water. Keeps hands up and above waist level.					
7. Dispenses another 5 mL of antimicrobial soap, and repeats the scrub.					
8. Washes for an additional 7 minutes without using a brush. Rinses so the contaminated water runs down the arms and off the elbows.					

297

Performance Criteria	*	Self	Peer	Instructor	Comments
9. Dries hands and arms with a sterile towel. Uses a patting motion and continues up the forearms.					
10. Keeps hands above waist before donning sterile gown.					
Additional Comments					

Total number of points possible _____

Total number of points received _____

Grade _____ *Instructor's initials* _____ *Date* _____

Performance Objective

By following a routine procedure that meets stated protocols, the student will be able to perform sterile gloving.

Evaluation and Grading Criteria

3   Student competently met the stated criteria without assistance.

2   Student required assistance in order to meet the stated criteria.

1   Student showed uncertainty when performing the stated criteria.

0   Student was not prepared and needs to repeat the step.

N/A   No evaluation of this step.

Instructor shall define grades for each point range earned upon completion of each performance-evaluated task.

Performance Standards

The minimum number of satisfactory performances required prior to final evaluation is _____.

Instructor shall identify by ∗ those steps considered critical. If step is missed or minimum competency is not met, the evaluated procedure fails and must be repeated.

Performance Criteria	∗	Self	Peer	Instructor	Comments
1. The glove package should have already been opened before the surgical scrub. Makes sure to touch only the inside of the package at this point.					
2. Gloves dominant hand first.					
3. Pulls the glove over the hand, touching only the folded cuff.					
4. With dominant hand gloved, slides forefingers under the cuff of the other glove.					
5. Pulls the glove up over other hand.					
6. Unrolls the cuff from gloves.					
Additional Comments					

Total number of points possible _____

Total number of points received _____

Grade _____ Instructor's initials _____ Date _____

Performance Objective

By following a routine procedure that meets stated protocols, when provided with information concerning the type of surgery, the tooth, and the anesthetics used, the student will prepare the setup, prepare the patient, and assist in a surgical procedure.

Evaluation and Grading Criteria

3   Student competently met the stated criteria without assistance.

2   Student required assistance in order to meet the stated criteria.

1   Student showed uncertainty when performing the stated criteria.

0   Student was not prepared and needs to repeat the step.

N/A   No evaluation of this step.

Instructor shall define grades for each point range earned on completion of each performance-evaluated task.

Performance Standards

The minimum number of satisfactory performances required before final evaluation is _____.

Instructor shall identify by * those steps considered critical. If step is missed or minimum competency is not met, the evaluated procedure fails and must be repeated.

Performance Criteria	*	Self	Peer	Instructor	Comment
Preparing the Treatment Room					
1. Prepares the treatment room.					
2. Keeps instruments in their sterile wraps until ready for use; if a surgical tray is preset, opens the tray and places a sterile towel over the instruments.					
3. Places the appropriate local anesthetic on the tray.					
4. Places the appropriate forceps on the tray.					
Preparing the Patient					
1. Seats the patient and positions a sterile patient drape or towel.					
2. Takes the patient's vital signs and records them in the patient's record.					
3. Adjusts the dental chair to the proper position.					
4. Stays with the patient until the dentist enters the treatment room.					

Performance Criteria	*	Self	Peer	Instructor	Comment
During the Surgical Procedure					
1. Places personal protective equipment according to the procedure.					
2. Maintains the chain of asepsis.					
3. Monitors vital signs.					
4. Aspirates and retracts as needed.					
5. Transfers and receives instruments as needed.					
6. Assists in suture placement as needed.					
7. Maintains a clear operating field with adequate light and irrigation.					
8. Steadies the patient's head and mandible if necessary.					
9. Observes the patient's condition and anticipates the dentist's needs.					
10. Provides postoperative instructions.					
11. Maintains patient comfort and follows appropriate infection control measures throughout the procedure.					
12. Documents procedure in patient record.					
Additional Comment					

Total number of points possible _____

Total number of points received _____

Grade _____ *Instructor's initials* _____ *Date* _____

Performance Objective

By following a routine procedure that meets stated protocols, the student will be able to assist in the placement of a suture.

Evaluation and Grading Criteria

3   Student competently met the stated criteria without assistance.

2   Student required assistance in order to meet the stated criteria.

1   Student showed uncertainty when performing the stated criteria.

0   Student was not prepared and needs to repeat the step.

N/A   No evaluation of this step.

Instructor shall define grades for each point range earned upon completion of each performance-evaluated task.

Performance Standards

The minimum number of satisfactory performances required prior to final evaluation is _____.

Instructor shall identify by ∗ those steps considered critical. If step is missed or minimum competency is not met, the evaluated procedure fails and must be repeated.

Performance Criteria	∗	Self	Peer	Instructor	Comments
1. Places personal protective equipment according to the procedure.					
2. Removes the suture material from its sterile package.					
3. Using the needle holder, clamps the suture needle at the upper third.					
4. Transfers the needle holder to the surgeon while grasping the hinge, allowing the surgeon to grasp the handle of the instrument.					
5. Retracts the tongue or cheek to provide a clear line of vision for the surgeon as the sutures are placed.					
6. After the tying of each suture, if directed by the surgeon, uses the suture scissors to cut the sutures, leaving approximately 2–3 mm of suture material beyond the knot.					
7. Retrieves the suturing supplies from the surgeon and replaces them on the surgical tray.					
8. Records the numbers and types of sutures placed in the patient's record.					
Additional Comments					

Total number of points possible _____

Total number of points received _____

Grade _____ *Instructor's initials* _____ *Date* _____

COMPETENCY 26-7 PERFORMING SUTURE REMOVAL (EXPANDED FUNCTION)

Performance Objective

By following a routine procedure that meets stated protocols, the student will be able to perform a suture removal.

Evaluation and Grading Criteria

3   Student competently met the stated criteria without assistance.

2   Student required assistance in order to meet the stated criteria.

1   Student showed uncertainty when performing the stated criteria.

0   Student was not prepared and needs to repeat the step.

N/A   No evaluation of this step.

Instructor shall define grades for each point range earned upon completion of each performance-evaluated task.

Performance Standards

The minimum number of satisfactory performances required prior to final evaluation is _____.

Instructor shall identify by * those steps considered critical. If step is missed or minimum competency is not met, the evaluated procedure fails and must be repeated.

Performance Criteria	*	Self	Peer	Instructor	Comments
1. Surgeon examines the surgical site to evaluate healing. If healing is satisfactory, the sutures can be removed.					
2. Instrument setup complete.					
3. Swabs the site with an antiseptic agent to remove any debris.					
4. Uses cotton pliers to hold the suture gently away from the tissue to expose the attachment of the knot. Slips one blade of the suture scissors gently under the suture. Cuts near the tissue.					
5. Uses cotton pliers to grasp the knot and gently tugs it so that the suture slides through the tissue.					
6. If there is bleeding, irrigates the surgical site with an antiseptic solution or warm saline solution. Applies a compress briefly to the surgical site to promote clotting.					
7. Counts the sutures that have been removed and compares the number with the number indicated on the patient's record.					
Additional Comments					

Total number of points possible _____

Total number of points received _____

Grade _____ *Instructor's initials* _____ *Date* _____

27 Pediatric Dentistry

TRUE/FALSE

_____ 1. Pediatric dentistry is the specialized area of dentistry limited to the care of patients from 6 months to 21 years of age.

_____ 2. Many pediatric dental offices are designed with several dental chairs arranged in one large treatment area or bay.

_____ 3. In the best interest of special needs patients, there dental care should be from an oral surgeon who has the appropriate education and training.

_____ 4. For any patient 19 years of age or younger, a parent or legal guardian must give his or her consent before any dental treatment can be provided.

_____ 5. Behavioral assessment is used to evaluate the communication skills of the patient and determine what behavior management techniques are necessary.

_____ 6. Prevention is one of the most encompassing areas for a pediatric dental practice.

_____ 7. Sealants are a common preventive procedure performed in a pediatric office.

_____ 8. The two matrix systems commonly placed on primary molar teeth are the clear Mylar strip and Universal band.

_____ 9. A gold crown would be the treatment of choice for a badly decayed primary molar.

_____ 10. A tooth that has been avulsed, means that it has been knocked completely out of the mouth.

MATCHING

Match the following pediatric procedures with their area of care:

_____ 11. Fluoride treatment

_____ 12. Class II amalgam filling

_____ 13. Pulpotomy

_____ 14. Space maintenance

_____ 15. Correcting a crossbite

A. Endodontic treatment

B. Interceptive orthodontics

C. Preventive care

D. Restorative dentistry

E. Preventive orthodontics

SHORT ANSWER

16. List the stages of behavior by age groups.

17. Describe the techniques to be used when introducing a child to a radiographic procedure.

INTERACTIVE DENTAL OFFICE PATIENT CASE EXERCISE

Access the *Interactive Dental Office on Evolve* and click on the patient case file for Raul Ortega, Jr.
- Review Raul's record.
- Answer the following questions:

1. What teeth are visible on the maxillary occlusal film taken on Raul?

2. Could the absence of fluoridated water be the reason for Raul's having baby bottle mouth syndrome?

3. What is the normal age range for the eruption of permanent first molars?

4. Would the placement of a stainless steel crown on Raul be considered an expanded function for the dental assistant?

5. Is the cement used for cementation of the stainless steel crown permanent or temporary?

COMPETENCY 27-1 ASSISTING IN PULPOTOMY OF A PRIMARY TOOTH

Performance Objective

By following a routine procedure that meets stated protocols, the student will be able to assist in the pulpotomy of a primary tooth.

Evaluation and Grading Criteria

3   Student competently met the stated criteria without assistance.

2   Student required assistance in order to meet the stated criteria.

1   Student showed uncertainty when performing the stated criteria.

0   Student was not prepared and needs to repeat the step.

N/A   No evaluation of this step.

Instructor shall define grades for each point range earned upon completion of each performance-evaluated task.

Performance Standards

The minimum number of satisfactory performances required prior to final evaluation is _____.

Instructor shall identify by * those steps considered critical. If step is missed or minimum competency is not met, the evaluated procedure fails and must be repeated.

Performance Criteria	*	Self	Peer	Instructor	Comments
1. Gathers the appropriate setup.					
2. Places personal protective equipment according to procedure.					
3. Assists in the administration of the local anesthetic agent.					
4. Places the dental dam.					
5. Assists the dentist using the air/water syringe and HVE while the dentist uses a round bur in the low-speed handpiece to remove the caries and expose the pulp chamber.					
6. Transfers instruments throughout the procedure.					
7. Prepares a sterile cotton pellet moistened with formocresol and transferred when needed.					
8. Once bleeding is controlled, mixes the zinc oxide–eugenol (ZOE) paste, for placement.					
9. Maintains patient comfort and follows appropriate infection control throughout the procedure.					
10. Documents procedure correctly.					
Additional Comments					

Total number of points possible _____

Total number of points received _____

Grade _____ Instructor's initials _____ Date _____

COMPETENCY 27-2 ASSISTING IN THE PLACEMENT OF A STAINLESS STEEL CROWN

Performance Objective

By following a routine procedure that meets stated protocols, the student will be able to assist in the placement of a stainless steel crown.

Evaluation and Grading Criteria

3   Student competently met the stated criteria without assistance.

2   Student required assistance in order to meet the stated criteria.

1   Student showed uncertainty when performing the stated criteria.

0   Student was not prepared and needs to repeat the step.

N/A   No evaluation of this step.

Instructor shall define grades for each point range earned upon completion of each performance-evaluated task.

Performance Standards

The minimum number of satisfactory performances required prior to final evaluation is _____.

Instructor shall identify by * those steps considered critical. If step is missed or minimum competency is not met, the evaluated procedure fails and must be repeated.

Performance Criteria	*	Self	Peer	Instructor	Comments
1. Gathers the appropriate setup.					
2. Places personal protective equipment according to procedure.					
Preparing the Tooth					
1. Assists in the administration of the local anesthetic.					
2. Places the dental dam or cotton rolls to isolate the tooth.					
3. The dentist uses the high-speed handpiece and a tapered diamond or carbide bur to prepare the tooth in a method similar to that for a cast crown (see Chapter 23).					
4. The dentist reduces the entire circumference of the tooth and the height of the tooth.					
5. All dental caries are removed with hand instruments and burs.					
Selecting and Sizing the Stainless Steel Crown					
1. Selects the crown and transfers it to the dentist to be tried on the prepared tooth.					
2. The stainless steel crown is properly sized when it fits snugly on the prepared tooth and has both mesial and distal contact.					
3. Cleans and sterilizes any crowns that were tried in the mouth but not used, then returns them to storage.					

Performance Criteria	*	Self	Peer	Instructor	Comments
Trimming and Contouring the Crown					
1. Readies the crown and bridge scissors for the dentist to use to reduce the height of the crown until it is approximately the same height as the adjacent teeth.					
2. Places a green stone on the high-speed handpiece for the dentist to smooth the rough edges of the crown along the cervical margin.					
3. Places a rubber wheel on the slow-speed handpiece for the dentist to polish the cervical margin of the crown.					
4. Readies articulating paper to check the occlusion and make adjustments as needed.					
5. Transfers contouring pliers to the dentist to crimp the cervical margins of the crown toward the tooth to obtain a tight fit and a proper cervical contour.					
Cementation					
1. Rinses and dries the tooth thoroughly. Places cotton rolls to maintain dry conditions.					
2. Mixes the permanent cement.					
3. Lines the crown with cement and transfers to the dentist for placement.					
4. Transfers an explorer to the dentist to remove the excess cement from around the tooth.					
5. Uses dental floss to remove any remaining cement from the interproximal areas.					
6. Uses the air-water syringe and high-volume evacuator tip to rinse the patient's mouth before dismissal.					
Additional Comments					

Total number of points possible _____

Total number of points received _____

Grade _____ Instructor's initials _____ Date _____

28 Orthodontics

TRUE/FALSE

_____ 1. Malocclusion is an abnormal or malpositioned relationship of the maxillary teeth to the mandibular teeth when occluded.

_____ 2. Motivation for seeking orthodontic treatment is not an essential factor.

_____ 3. One objective in the orthodontic exam is to evaluate the facial symmetry.

_____ 4. There are four standard extraoral photographs taken during the clinical examination.

_____ 5. Fixed appliances in orthodontics are commonly known as braces.

_____ 6. The radiographic image routinely exposed in orthodontics is the panoramic exposure.

_____ 7. Brackets are bonded to the mesial and distal surface of anterior and premolar teeth.

_____ 8. A week prior to the banding appointment, a separator is placed interproximal to open the mesial and distal spaces of the tooth slightly for easier seating of the band.

_____ 9. Throughout a patient's orthodontic treatment, it is recommended that soft foods should be avoided to prevent dislodging the brackets and bands.

_____ 10. A loose band can be the result of a break in the cement seal or from poor food choices.

MATCHING

Match each instrument with its use.

_____ 11. Aids in seating a molar band   A. Distal end cutter

_____ 12. Tucks the twisted ligature tie under the arch wire   B. Weingart pliers

_____ 13. Cuts the end of the arch wire   C. Bite stick

_____ 14. Used in placing the arch wire in the brackets   D. Ligature director

_____ 15. Helps form and bend wires   E. Bird-beak pliers

Match the component of braces with its description.

_____ 16. Holds the end of the arch wire and additional power products   A. Bracket

_____ 17. Holds the arch wire in place within the bracket   B. Arch wire

   C. Separator

_____ 18. Creates tooth movement   D. Ligature tie

_____ 19. Attachment for the arch wire   E. Molar band

_____ 20. Creates space to seat bands

SHORT ANSWER

21. What are the three major diagnostic implements used to make a diagnosis and prepare a treatment plan?

22. At each adjustment appointment, it is the responsibility of the chairside assistant to evaluate the patient's appliance. What specific things should the assistant look for?

Access the *Interactive Dental Office on Evolve* and click on the patient case file for Kevin McClelland.
- Review Kevin's record.
- Complete all exercises on Evolve for Kevin's case.
- Answer the following questions:

1. Looking at Kevin's panoramic, which teeth are banded?

2. What types of ligatures are used for Kevin's orthodontic treatment?

3. The bands have labial hooks. What are these used for?

4. What type of oral hygiene instructions should be provided to Kevin while orthodontic treatment is in progress?

5. Kevin is scheduled to have a sealant placed on tooth #19. Can a sealant be placed while Kevin is receiving orthodontic treatment?

COMPETENCY 28-1 PLACING AND REMOVING ELASTOMERIC RING SEPARATORS (EXPANDED FUNCTION)

Performance Objective

By following a routine procedure that meets stated protocols, the student will be able to place and remove elastomeric ring separators.

Evaluation and Grading Criteria

3   Student competently met the stated criteria without assistance.

2   Student required assistance in order to meet the stated criteria.

1   Student showed uncertainty when performing the stated criteria.

0   Student was not prepared and needs to repeat the step.

N/A   No evaluation of this step.

Instructor shall define grades for each point range earned upon completion of each performance-evaluated task.

Performance Standards

The minimum number of satisfactory performances required prior to final evaluation is _____.

Instructor shall identify by ∗ those steps considered critical. If step is missed or minimum competency is not met, the evaluated procedure fails and must be repeated.

Performance Criteria	∗	Self	Peer	Instructor	Comments
1. Gathers the appropriate setup.					
2. Explains the procedure to the patient.					
3. Places personal protective equipment according to procedure.					
Placing Elastomeric Ring Separators					
1. Places the separator over the beaks of separating pliers.					
2. Stretches the ring and then uses a seesaw motion to gently force it through the proximal contact.					
3. An alternative method is to use two loops of dental floss to stretch the ring and guide it into place.					
4. Leaves this type of separator in place for up to 2 weeks.					
Removing Elastomeric Ring Separators					
1. Slides an orthodontic scaler into the doughnut-shaped separator.					
2. Uses slight pressure to remove the ring from under the contact.					
Additional Comments					

Total number of points possible _____

Total number of points received _____

Grade _____ Instructor's initials _____ Date _____

315

COMPETENCY 28-2 ASSISTING IN THE FITTING AND CEMENTATION OF ORTHODONTIC BANDS

Performance Objective

By following a routine procedure that meets stated protocols, the student will be able to assist in the fitting and cementation of orthodontic bands.

Evaluation and Grading Criteria

3   Student competently met the stated criteria without assistance.

2   Student required assistance in order to meet the stated criteria.

1   Student showed uncertainty when performing the stated criteria.

0   Student was not prepared and needs to repeat the step.

N/A   No evaluation of this step.

Instructor shall define grades for each point range earned upon completion of each performance-evaluated task.

Performance Standards

The minimum number of satisfactory performances required prior to final evaluation is _____.

Instructor shall identify by * those steps considered critical. If step is missed or minimum competency is not met, the evaluated procedure fails and must be repeated.

Performance Criteria	*	Self	Peer	Instructor	Comments
1. Gathers the appropriate setup.					
2. Places personal protective equipment according to procedure.					
Preparation 1. Places each preselected orthodontic band on a small square of masking tape, with the occlusal surface on the tape and the gingival margin of the band upright.					
2. Wipes any buccal tubes or attachments with ChapStick or utility wax.					
Mixing and Placing the Cement 1. The teeth are isolated and dried.					
2. At a signal from the orthodontist, dispenses the cement according to the manufacturer's directions, then quickly mixes the cement until it is homogeneous.					
3. Holds the band by the margin of the masking tape. The gingival surface is upright, and the cement spatula is placed on the margin of the band.					
4. Wipes the spatula over the margin, allowing the cement to flow into the circumference of the band.					
5. Transfers the cement-filled band to the orthodontist, who inverts the band over the tooth.					
6. Transfers the band seater to the orthodontist, who places it on the buccal margin of the band.					
7. Instructs the patient to bite gently on the band.					

317

Performance Criteria	*	Self	Peer	Instructor	Comments
8. Excess cement is forced out from under the gingival and occlusal margins of the bands and is allowed to harden.					
9. The process is repeated until all of the bands are seated.					
Removing Excess Cement 1. After the cement has reached its final stage of setting, a scaler or explorer is used to remove the excess cement on the enamel surfaces.					
2. The patient's mouth is rinsed, flossed, and checked to ensure that all of the excess cement has been removed.					
3. Documents procedure in patient record.					
Additional Comments					

Total number of points possible _____

Total number of points received _____

Grade _____ *Instructor's initials* _____ *Date* _____

COMPETENCY 28-3 ASSISTING IN THE DIRECT BONDING OF ORTHODONTIC BRACKETS

Performance Objective

By following a routine procedure that meets stated protocols, the student will be able to assist in the direct bonding of orthodontic brackets.

Evaluation and Grading Criteria

3	Student competently met the stated criteria without assistance.
2	Student required assistance in order to meet the stated criteria.
1	Student showed uncertainty when performing the stated criteria.
0	Student was not prepared and needs to repeat the step.
N/A	No evaluation of this step.

Instructor shall define grades for each point range earned upon completion of each performance-evaluated task.

Performance Standards

The minimum number of satisfactory performances required prior to final evaluation is _____.

Instructor shall identify by * those steps considered critical. If step is missed or minimum competency is not met, the evaluated procedure fails and must be repeated.

Performance Criteria	*	Self	Peer	Instructor	Comments
1. Gathers the appropriate setup.					
2. Places personal protective equipment according to the procedure.					
Preparing the Teeth					
1. Cleans the tooth surface with prophy cup and pumice slurry and then rinses and dries teeth.					
2. Uses either cotton rolls or retractors to isolate the teeth.					
3. An etchant gel is placed on the facial area of the tooth that is to receive bonding. This remains on the tooth for the manufacturer's specified time, which is then rinsed and dried thoroughly.					
Bonding the Brackets					
1. The orthodontist applies a liquid resin to the prepared tooth surface.					
2. Mixes a small quantity of bonding material and places it on the back of the bracket. Uses bracket placement tweezers to transfer the bracket to the orthodontist.					
3. Transfers the orthodontic scaler. The orthodontist places the bracket and moves it into final position with a scaler.					

Performance Criteria	*	Self	Peer	Instructor	Comments
4. The orthodontist uses the scaler to immediately remove the excess bonding material before light-curing the material.					
5. Procedure documented in patient record.					
Additional Comments					

Total number of points possible _____

Total number of points received _____

Grade _____ *Instructor's initials* _____ *Date* _____

COMPETENCIES 28-4 AND 28-5 PLACING AND REMOVING ARCH WIRES AND TIES (EXPANDED FUNCTION)

Performance Objective

By following a routine procedure that meets stated protocols, the student will demonstrate the proper technique for placing and removing ligature wires and elastomeric ties.

Evaluation and Grading Criteria

3	Student competently met the stated criteria without assistance.
2	Student required assistance in order to meet the stated criteria.
1	Student showed uncertainty when performing the stated criteria.
0	Student was not prepared and needs to repeat the step.
N/A	No evaluation of this step.

Instructor shall define grades for each point range earned on completion of each performance-evaluated task.

Performance Standards

The minimum number of satisfactory performances required before final evaluation is _____.

Instructor shall identify by * those steps considered critical. If step is missed or minimum competency is not met, the evaluated procedure fails and must be repeated.

Performance Criteria	*	Self	Peer	Instructor	Comment
Placing the Arch Wires					
1. Gathers the appropriate setup.					
2. Places personal protective equipment according to procedure.					
3. Wire premeasured before placed in the mouth.					
4. If additional bends are needed, transfers appropriate plier to orthodontist.					
5. Centers arch wire.					
6. Distal ends of wire placed in buccal tube with correct length.					
Placing the Ligature Wires					
7. Places the ligature wire around the bracket and uses the ligature director to push the wire against the tie wing.					
8. Uses the hemostat to twist the wire snugly against the bracket; repeats the procedure until all brackets were ligated.					
9. Uses a ligature cutter to cut the excess wire, leaving a 4- to 5-mm pigtail.					
10. Tucks the pigtails under the arch wire using the correct instruments.					
11. Wire is not protruding to injure the patient.					

321

Performance Criteria	*	Self	Peer	Instructor	Comment
Removing the Ligature Wire					
1. Holds the ligature cutter properly and uses the beaks of the pliers to cut the wire at the easiest access.					
2. Carefully unwraps the ligature and removes it.					
3. Does not twist or pull as the ligatures are cut and removed.					
4. Continues cutting and removing until all brackets are untied.					
5. Maintains patient comfort and follows appropriate infection control measures throughout the procedure.					
Placing the Elastomeric Tie					
1. Gathered the appropriate setup.					
2. Uses a hemostat and places the beaks of the pliers on a tie, then locks the pliers.					
3. Places the tie on the gingival portion of one tie wing and slips the tie around the edges of the bracket.					
4. Releases the pliers.					
Removing the Elastomeric Tie					
1. Uses the orthodontic scaler held in a pen grasp and supports the teeth and tissue with the other hand.					
2. Places the scaler tie between the bracket and tie wings and pulls the tie at the gingival position with a rolling motion.					
3. Removes the tie in an occlusal direction.					
4. Maintains patient comfort and follows appropriate infection control measures throughout the procedure.					
5. Documents procedure in patient record.					
Additional Comments					

Total number of points possible _____

Total number of points received _____

Grade _____ Instructor's initials _____ Date _____

29 Employment

TRUE/FALSE

_____ 1. The dental assistant is major part of the dental team and should have pride and self-fulfillment when joining a private practice.

_____ 2. Dental insurance companies hire dental assistants with knowledge of processing dental claims and customer service.

_____ 3. Your first contact with a prospective employer will most likely be by email.

_____ 4. Social media is an extremely powerful tool when searching for employment opportunities.

_____ 5. A résumé communicates a minimum amount of information through a maximum number of words.

_____ 6. There is only one correct way to write a résumé.

_____ 7. Your résumé should include your most recent employment to your least recent employment experiences.

_____ 8. CPR would be considered a certification that should be listed on your résumé.

_____ 9. Volunteer work isn't important to list on your résumé because it does not pertain to dentistry.

_____ 10. It is best to plan to arrive 15 minutes before the scheduled time of an interview.

SHORT ANSWER

11. Name the various career opportunities that a dental assistant can pursue.

12. Name the major professional networking site.

13. Give 10 tips for having a good interview.

323

COMPETENCY 29-1 PREPARING A PROFESSIONAL RÉSUMÉ

Performance Objective

By following a routine procedure that meets stated protocols, the student will be able to prepare a résumé to be used for seeking employment.

Evaluation and Grading Criteria

3	Student competently met the stated criteria without assistance.
2	Student required assistance in order to meet the stated criteria.
1	Student showed uncertainty when performing the stated criteria.
0	Student was not prepared and needs to repeat the step.
N/A	No evaluation of this step.

Instructor shall define grades for each point range earned upon completion of each performance-evaluated task.

Performance Standards

The minimum number of satisfactory performances required prior to final evaluation is _____.

Instructor shall identify by * those steps considered critical. If step is missed or minimum competency is not met, the evaluated procedure fails and must be repeated.

Performance Criteria	*	Self	Peer	Instructor	Comments
1. Keeps the résumé to one page.					
2. Uses a standard 8½ × 11-inch white or ivory rag paper.					
3. Uses common typefaces.					
4. Uses 1-inch margins on all sides.					
5. Uses a 12-point font size.					
6. Ensures that the résumé is neat and error free.					
7. Makes the résumé concise and easy to read.					
Additional Comments					

Total number of points possible _____

Total number of points received _____

Grade _____ Instructor's initials _____ Date _____

Bones of the Skull

Describe the location of the following cranial bones:

1. Frontal
2. Temporal
3. Parietal
4. Sphenoid
5. Occipital
6. Ethmoid

Types of Teeth

Describe the location and function of the four types of teeth:

1. Incisors
2. Canines
3. Premolars
4. Molars

Bones of the Face

Describe the location of the following facial bones:

1. Zygomatic
2. Nasal
3. Inferior con-
   chae
4. Maxillary
5. Lacrimal
6. Mandible
7. Palatine
8. Vomer

Surfaces of Teeth

Describe the surface location of the six types of teeth:

1. Facial
2. Lingual
3. Occlusal
4. Incisal
5. Mesial
6. Distal

Tissues of the Teeth

Identify the four tissues of the teeth and their makeup.

Tooth Eruption

Describe the age of eruption for the following permanent maxillary and mandibular teeth:

1. Central incisors
2. Canines
3. Second premolars
4. Second molars
5. Lateral incisors
6. First premolars
7. First molars
8. Third molars

Bones of the Skull

1. Forehead
2. Sides
3. Roof
4. Anterior base
5. Base
6. Orbit and floor

Types of Teeth

1. Front of mouth/cutting food
2. Corner of mouth/cutting and tearing
3. Back of mouth/grasping and tearing
4. Back of mouth/chewing and grinding

Bones of the Face

1. Cheeks
2. Nose
3. Interior nose
4. Upper jaw
5. Orbit
6. Lower jaw
7. Hard palate
8. Base of nose

Surfaces of Teeth

1. Toward the lips
2. Toward the tongue
3. Back chewing surface
4. Front chewing surface
5. Interproximal surface closest to midline
6. Interproximal surface away from midline

Tissues of the Teeth

1. Enamel—the outer covering of the coronal portion of the tooth
2. Dentin—makes up most of the tooth and is reparative
3. Cementum—the outer layer of the root structure for attachment
4. Pulp—contains the nerves and blood of the tooth

Tooth Eruption

1. 6–8 years
2. 9–12 years
3. 10–13 years
4. 11–13 years
5. 7–9 years
6. 10–11 years
7. 6–17 years
8. 17–21 years

Emergency Preparedness

Describe the roles of each professional in an emergency situation:

1. Calls emergency services and remains on the phone

2. Chairside assistant

3. Dentist

Emergency Situation

How would you respond to a patient with syncope?

Emergency Situation

How would you respond to a patient with hypoglycemia?

Cardiopulmonary Resuscitation

Define *CAB* of CPR.

Emergency Drugs

The following drugs can be found in an emergency kit. For what emergency is each drug prepared?

1. Epinephrine   4. Nitroglycerin

2. Antihistamine   5. Inhaler

3. Diazepam   6. Ammonia inhalant

Emergency Situation

How would you respond to a patient with anaphylaxis?

Emergency Preparedness

1. Calls emergency services.

2. Retrieves oxygen/drug kit and assesses patient.

3. Remains with patient and determines patient needs.

Emergency Situation

1. Place patient in supine position.

2. Prepare ammonia inhalant.

3. Prepare oxygen if needed.

4. Monitor and record vital signs.

Emergency Situation

1. Position patient in supine position.

2. Prepare epinephrine for administration.

3. Prepare for CPR if needed.

4. Monitor and record vital signs.

Emergency Situation

1. Administer concentrated sugar under patient's tongue.

2. Prepare for CPR if needed.

3. Monitor and record vital signs.

Cardiopulmonary Resuscitation

C = Compressions - Push hard and fast on the center of the victim's chest

A = Airway - Tilt the victim's head back and lift the chin to open the airway

B = Breathing - Give mouth-to-mouth rescue breathing

Emergency Drugs

1. Acute allergic reaction

2. Allergic response

3. Seizure

4. Chest pain

5. Asthma attacks

6. Syncope

Disease Transmission

Describe the following methods of disease transmission:

1. Direct   4. Airborne

2. Indirect   5. Dental unit waterlines

3. Splash/splatter

Disinfection Procedures

1. Define disinfection.

2. Describe the spray-wipe-spray technique.

Diseases of Major Concern

Describe the following diseases and their effects:

1. Hepatitis B

2. Human immunodeficiency virus infection

3. Tuberculosis

Sterilization Procedures

Describe the following sterilization methods:

1. Steam sterilization

2. Chemical vapor sterilization

3. Dry-heat sterilization

Personal Protective Equipment

What are the four components of PPE, and how do they protect the caregiver?

Hazard Communication

Describe the following parts of a hazard communication program:

1. Written program   4. Labeling

2. Chemical inventory   5. Training

3. SDS

Disease Transmission

1. Contact with infectious lesions

2. Contact with a contaminated object

3. Exposure to blood, saliva, and body fluids

4. Microorganisms in sprays, mists, and aerosols

5. Microorganisms in water from dental unit

Diseases of Major Concern

1. Bloodborne viral infection that affects the liver and is transmitted by body fluids

2. Bloodborne viral infection that affects the immune system and is transmitted by body fluids

3. Bacterial infection that mostly affects the lungs

Personal Protective Equipment

1. Protective clothing protects the skin and underclothing from exposure.

2. A protective mask prevents the inhalation of infectious organisms.

3. Protective eyewear protects the eye from aerosol and debris.

4. Protective gloves prevent direct contact with contaminated objects.

Disinfection Procedures

1. Killing or inhibiting pathogens from growth by the use of a chemical agent

2. Spray—Thoroughly spray the surface.

3. Wipe—Wipe the surface clean.

4. Spray—Spray with disinfectant for recommended time.

Sterilization Procedures

1. Superheated steam under pressure for a recommended time (250°F, 20 minutes, 15–20 psi)

2. Superheated chemical under pressure for a recommended time(270°F, 20–40 minutes, 20 psi)

3. Superheat with no moisture or chemical for a recommended time (340°F, 60 minutes)

Hazard Communication

1. Documentation maintained to identify employees who are exposed to hazardous materials

2. Comprehensive list of chemicals used in the dental office

3. Information by the manufacturer describing the physical and chemical properties of a product

4. All containers labeled with name of product and any hazardous material

5. Training required for (1) new employees, (2) when a new chemical is acquired, and (3) yearly for continuing education

Radiation Protection

1. Define three types of radiation protection methods for the patient.

2. Define two types of radiation protection methods for the operator.

Processing Radiographs

1. Describe the role of developer in the processing of exposed radiographs.

2. Describe the role of fixer in the processing of exposed radiographs.

Concept of Paralleling Technique

Describe the positioning of the film/sensor, tooth, and central ray for the paralleling technique.

Technique Errors

Describe how the following errors occur:

1. Elongation
2. Overlapping
3. Underexposure
4. Cone cutting
5. Foreshortening
6. Herringbone pattern
7. Double exposure
8. Bent film

Concept of Bisecting Technique

Describe the positioning of the film/sensor, tooth, and central ray for the bisecting technique.

Types of Extraoral Films

Define the use for the following extraoral films:

1. Panoramic
2. Cephalometric
3. Tomogram

Radiation Protection

1. Proper film/sensor-exposure technique Use of film/sensor-holding instruments Lead apron and thyroid collar

2. Personnel monitoring Equipment monitoring

Concept of Paralleling Technique

The x-ray beam is directed to the right angle of the film/sensor and the long axis of the tooth.

Concept of Bisecting Technique

The film is angled to the long axis of the tooth.

The space between the film and tooth is bisected.

The x-ray beam is directed perpendicular to the bisecting line.

Processing Radiographs

1. Developer reacts with silver halide crystals on the film that were affected by radiation. These crystals form the images.

2. Fixer removes any crystals that did not react, hardens the emulsion, and preserves the image.

Technique Errors

1. Not enough vertical angulation

2. Central ray not directed through interproximal space

3. Settings too low

4. X-ray beam did not expose entire film

5. Too much vertical angulation

6. Film reversed

7. Film exposed twice

8. Film bent in mouth

Types of Extraoral Films

1. Provides a view of the entire maxilla and mandible

2. Provides a lateral view of the skull

3. Provides a view of sections of the temporomandibular joint (TMJ)

Hand Cutting Instruments

Define the use for the following instruments:

1. Excavator
2. Hatchet
3. Hoe
4. Chisel
5. Gingival margin trimer

Endodontic Instruments

Define the use for the following instruments:

1. Broach
2. File
3. Rubber stopper
4. Endodontic explorer
5. Spreader
6. Plugger

Restorative Instruments

Define the use for the following instruments:

1. Amalgam carrier
2. Amalgam condenser
3. Burnisher
4. Discoid-cleoid carver
5. Hollenback carver
6. Composite instrument

Oral Surgery Instruments

Define the use for the following instruments:

1. Elevator
2. Forceps
3. Surgical curette
4. Rongeur
5. Bone file
6. Scalpel
7. Hemostat
8. Needle holder

Handpiece and Rotary Instruments

Define the use for the following instruments:

1. High-speed handpiece
2. Low-speed handpiece
3. Straight attachment
4. Contra-angle attachment
5. Friction-grip bur
6. Latch-type bur

Orthodontic Instruments

Define the use for the following instruments:

1. Ligature director
2. Band plugger
3. Bite stick
4. Bird-beak pliers
5. Distal end cutter
6. Pin and ligature cutter
7. Band remover
8. Howe pliers

Hand Cutting Instruments

1. To remove decay and debris from a cavity preparation
2. To smooth the walls and floors of a prepared tooth
3. To smooth the floors of a prepared tooth
4. To smooth the enamel margin, and form sharp lines, point angles, and retention grooves
5. To place bevels along the gingival margin

Restorative Instruments

1. To carry amalgam to the prepared tooth
2. To pack amalgam into the tooth
3. To smooth amalgam
4. To carve the occlusal anatomy of amalgam
5. To carve the interproximal anatomy of amalgam
6. To place composite material into the prepared tooth

Handpiece and Rotary Instruments

1. Runs at 450,000 rpm to remove decay and large amount of tooth structure
2. Runs at 25,000 rpm to finish, contour, and polish
3. Fits on low-speed handpiece and holds long-shank lab burs
4. Fits on low-speed handpiece, and holds latch-type burs, prophy cups, and brushes
5. Available in assorted shapes and fits on high-speed handpiece
6. Available in assorted shapes and fits on contra-angle of low-speed handpiece

Endodontic Instruments

1. To remove pulp tissue
2. To smooth and enlarge the canal
3. Small piece of rubber to measure the length of the file
4. Long and straight explorer to locate canal openings
5. Pointed end to assist in filling the canal
6. Flat end to assist in filling the canal

Oral Surgery Instruments

1. To reflect and retract the periosteum from the bone
2. To remove the tooth from the socket
3. To clean and remove diseased tissue from the socket
4. To trim alveolar bone
5. To smooth the surface of the bone
6. Surgical knife
7. To grasp and hold items
8. To hold the surgical needle firmly during suturing

Orthodontic Instruments

1. To guide and tuck ligature ties under the arch wire
2. To aid in seating molar bands
3. To aid in seating molar bands
4. To form and bend the arch wire
5. To cut and hold the end of the arch wire
6. To cut ligature wire
7. To remove bands
8. Versatile pliers used to bend wires

Preventive Materials

Describe the following preventive materials and their use:

1. Systemic fluoride

2. Topical fluoride

3. Sealants

Impression Materials

Describe the following impression materials and their use:

1. Hydrocolloids

2. Reversible hydrocolloids

3. Elastomeric

Laboratory Procedures

Describe the following procedures completed in the dental laboratory:

1. Diagnostic cast

2. Custom tray

3. Provisional crown

4. Vacuum-formed tray

Amalgam

Describe the makeup of amalgam.

Composite Resin

Describe the makeup of composite resin.

Cements

Identify the use for the following cements:

1. Glass ionomer

2. Zinc phosphate

3. Zinc oxide–eugenol

4. Polycarboxylate

5. Intermediate restorative material

Amalgam

Silver (to strengthen)

Tin (to strengthen, and for workability)

Copper (to strengthen, and for low corrosive properties)

Mercury (to provide easy application and adaptability to tooth structure)

Composite Resin

Resin matrix (also known as BIS-GMA, a material used to make synthetic resins)

Inorganic fillers (quartz, glass, silica)

Coupling agent (to strengthen and chemically bond the filler to the resin matrix)

Cements

1. Permanent cementation, restorations, liners, and bonding

2. Permanent cementation and insulating base

3. Permanent cementation, temporary cementation, and insulating base

4. Permanent cementation and insulating base

5. Temporary restorative material

Preventive Materials

1. Mineral found in water, food, and supplements to prevent decay

2. Mineral found in toothpaste, mouth rinses, concentrated gel, and foam to prevent decay

3. Liquid resin applied and cured in the pits and fissures of teeth to prevent decay

Impression Materials

1. Referred to as alginate; used to obtain preliminary impressions for diagnostic purposes

2. Type of impression material with the ability to change its physical state

3. Referred to as a final impression; these materials get the most accurate impression

Laboratory Procedures

1. To diagnose, to fabricate an appliance, and for records

2. Type of tray that is fabricated specifically for a patient's mouth

3. Temporary coverage of a tooth or teeth made from acrylic or prefabricated material

4. Light-gauge plastic material that is form-fitted over a cast and then trimmed to fit over a patient arch

Preventive Procedures

Define the following procedures:

1. Flossing   3. Coronal polishing

2. Toothbrushing   4. Fluoride treatment

Oral Surgery

Define the following procedures:

1. Forceps extraction   4. Suture

2. Surgical impaction   5. Biopsy

3. Alveoloplasty

Restorative Classifications

Define the following cavity classifications:

1. Class I restorations   4. Class IV restorations

2. Class II restorations   5. Class V restorations

3. Class III restorations   6. Class VI restorations

Endodontics

Define the following procedures:

1. Indirect pulp capping   4. Pulpectomy

2. Direct pulp capping   5. Apicoectomy

3. Pulpotomy

Prosthodontics

Define the following procedures:

1. Inlay   5. Fixed bridge

2. Onlay   6. Partial denture

3. Veneer   7. Full denture

4. Crown

Periodontics

Define the following procedures:

1. Scaling   4. Gingivectomy

2. Root planing   5. Gingivoplasty

3. Gingival curettage   6. Osteoplasty

Preventive Procedures

1. To remove plaque from interproximal tooth surfaces
2. To remove plaque from tooth surfaces
3. To remove plaque and stains from teeth after calculus is removed
4. To apply topical fluoride to clean teeth

Restorative Classifications

1. Pit-and-fissure cavities
2. Posterior interproximal cavities
3. Anterior interproximal cavities
4. Anterior interproximal cavities involving the incisal edge
5. Smooth-surface cavities
6. Cavities or abrasions involving the incisal edge or occlusal cusp

Prosthodontics

1. Fixed restoration involving a portion of the occlusal and interproximal surface
2. Fixed restoration involving most of the occlusal and interproximal surface
3. Thin-shelled, tooth-colored restoration for facial surfaces
4. Fixed restoration covering all of the anatomic crown of a tooth
5. Fixed restoration replacing one or more teeth in the same arch
6. Removable prosthesis replacing one or more teeth in the same arch
7. Removable prosthesis replacing all teeth in the same arch

Oral Surgery

1. Removal of a fully erupted tooth
2. Removal of a tooth partially or totally covered by tissue and bone
3. Surgical contour of the bone and soft tissue after an extraction
4. Application of a material to control bleeding and promote healing
5. Surgical removal of tissue for analysis

Endodontics

1. Application of calcium hydroxide when the dental pulp is not exposed
2. Application of calcium hydroxide when the dental pulp has a slight exposure
3. Partial removal of the dental pulp
4. Complete removal of the dental pulp
5. Surgical removal of the apical portion of the root

Periodontics

1. Removal of calculus from a tooth surface
2. Removal of calculus and necrotic cementum
3. Removal of necrotic tissue from the gingival wall of the periodontal pocket
4. Surgical removal of diseased gingiva
5. Surgical reshaping of the gingival tissues
6. Surgical reshaping of bone